Tantric Sex

Emil Rachuean

Tantric Sex

A practical guide to physical pleasure

Astrolog Publishing House Ltd.

ISBN 965-494-180-5

© Astrolog Publishing House Ltd. 2003

P.O. Box 1123, Hod Hasharon 45111, Israel
Tel: 972-9-7412044
Fax: 972-9-7442714

10 9 8 7 6 5 4 3 2 1

Table of contents

Chapter 1

Tantric sex

What is tantric sex, and how is it different than any other kind of sex?

1

There are two central and essential principles in tantric sex. The first is the emphasis on and the importance of the woman's sexual fulfillment, and the second is the man's need to control ejaculation.

2

The word tantra is originally an Indian word that means "written text." A tantra is the written equivalent of the spoken or sung version that is known as a mantra, which is mainly used as a basis for meditation.

3

The best known tantric texts are *The Kama Sutra*, the *Ananga Ranga* and the *Kama Shastra* – three ancient Indian erotic manuals – as well as *The Perfumed Garden* and *The Pleasure Garden*, which are Arab studies of sexual techniques and moral faith, which were written at the beginning of the 17th century.

4

Unfortunately, the Tantra sources are shrouded in the mists of time, a great deal of which has passed since the ancient tantric studies first began. However, there are people who believe that Tantra has been propelling its students into the realms of sexual ecstasy for the last 5,000 years.

5

It seems that the roots of Tantra originated in India, in Hinduism, and from there it spread to Tibet, China, Nepal, Japan and South East Asia. As a result of its broad dissemination in the world, tantric symbols can be found in almost every ancient culture, including pictures from the Stone Age, Sumerian etchings, Egyptian texts, Hebrew writings, mystical Greek texts and Arab love poems.

6

The golden age of Tantra was apparently during the 11th and 12th centuries AD, when it was widely practiced in

India. Disaster struck in the 13th century, when the Moslem invasion brought about the destruction of the tantric writings and the execution of many tantrists. The movement sought safety by going underground (where most of it remained since those early times), and the practice of Tantra was mainly carried out in secret.

7

Actually, there are several different forms of Tantra, depending on the country in which it is practiced and the prevailing belief there. There are tantric Buddhists, who follow the Asiatic Buddhist faith. There are tantric Hindus, who follow the Hindu method with its rituals and belief in reincarnation. There are tantric Taoists, who follow the ancient Chinese philosophy in which the individual is directed to find and maintain a maximal level of inner energy, thereby achieving a state of harmony and union with the universe. And there are even tantric agnostics, who believe that nothing is known for certain, not even the existence of God.

8

In conclusion, tantric sex extracts the best from all the techniques found in these ancient cultures. It offers ways of improving lovemaking, and it permits the sexual focus to be shifted from the solely physical to the spiritual.

Chapter 2

Energy

*Sexual energy can be aroused,
guided and channeled*

1

Sexual energy can be aroused, guided and channeled in order to increase our health and our spirituality, thereby reaching the peak of perfection of Tantra, or celestial union. For Tantra practitioners, sex is not just a matter of pleasure, but a deep and basic approach to exchanges of energy.

A large part of the tantric belief relates to energy (prana to the Indians and chi to the Chinese), that is, to the way in which energy can change its focus. Tantra perceives sexual energy to be the strongest energy that exists, and proposes that it be used as a way to heighten sensitivity, achieve release from the limitations of the individual's life and attain the highest levels of ecstasy.

2

Sex, more than anything else, is a question of energy. Sexual energy flows through our bodies, according to the ancient tantric belief, like a powerful current of electricity. We are born with this energy just as we are born with the other parts of our body such as our internal organs or our ability to feel, breathe or speak. In other words, sexual energy is inside us, within reach, and is ready for us to use judiciously when we so wish. The essence of sexuality is found in this energy, so in order to find the true path to sexual happiness, this important current must be opened and activated.

Energy flows through the body in a series of complex paths or meridians. These paths are invisible, but their geography is mapped out in the tantric doctrine.

3

Sexual energy is powerful and can be directed beyond the sexual organs (where the main concentration of it is), that is, to the head and to the heart.

This possibility offers us an opportunity to undergo a completely new experience, an experience in which the energy rises up beyond the borders of the physical body. In this way, sex is elevated to another plane and becomes a means of attaining fierce joy and inner serenity (for which we all yearn) that will cause a wonderful revolution in our lives. By experiencing marvelous and fulfilling sex on a regular basis, we can become fully rounded people.

You may never have thought about tantric sex, but the topic is certainly worth examining in depth. Tantric sex helps many people turn something that was always good into something that is much better and much more wonderful. It requires time and practice, but, as we said above, it's certainly worth it.

Tantra is not an easy concept for Westerners, but after the first barriers – the perceptual and conceptual barriers – are removed, it is very easy for people to keep on practicing it, since sex serves as a natural source of powerful pleasure that is experienced by most people.

Ultimately, tantric sex means very different things to different people. Whether it aims at cosmic illumination or better sex, tantric sex has a great deal to offer and it can contribute tremendously to our everyday lives.

4

As we know, most of us consider this pleasure to be completely physical, and Tantra has a lot to teach us about this point. Tantra enables the person to rise above pure physicality and achieve a state of blessed happiness in which time and place are meaningless. In an extreme manner, it is possible to feel union with the universe as well as achieve cosmic illumination.

As we said, a good sex life exerts an enormous influence on us. In addition, it increases our chances of a long, healthy and happy life. This point of view offers a completely new perception regarding the art of making love. The tantric approach to sexual experiences may point the way to a longer, happier, fuller and more spiritual life.

5

In good sex, it is very important for each member of the couple to find a way to tune into the other person's energy, and, of course, to respond to this accordingly. The idea of energy exchanges during sex may sound odd to Westerners, but these energy exchanges are extremely important in the tantric belief and occur on a permanent basis; in other words, you will carry it with you forever. This means that you will always carry all the energy that has been given to you by your previous lovers, and if your sexual experience has been brief, unfulfilling or unhappy, you will carry this negative energy with you and exchange it with your future lovers.

Sexual energies are created and become harmonious mainly in certain sexual positions, in which the partners complete a circle of love by joining certain organs of their bodies such as their mouths, their tongues, their hands or even their feet. This promotes emotional closeness between two people and produces a feeling of togetherness, to the point (in extreme cases) that they feel that they have achieved perfect union.

6

That is another reason to ensure that all of your sexual experiences occur in a loving and stable relationship. Who said that Tantra is a license for sexual promiscuity in which love is completely unimportant? Tantra is actually the most moral viewpoint, and all the tantric texts assume that sex that is not performed in the framework of a loving relationship is nothing more than "second-rate sex."

7

Tantra is the philosophy of union, or perfection, and in order to achieve it, everything is considered an opportunity to learn and to add to the totality of human experience. One of the central tantric beliefs states that Tantra embraces opposites in which it does not see contradictions, but rather perfect matches for the sake of the creation of a whole.

For this reason, a man and a woman are not perceived as opposites facing each other, but rather as two complementary factors who need each other and who meet up in every human being. Each one, whether a man or a woman, is considered to possess both male and female characteristics.

Therefore, according to the tantric belief, it is essential to take another step forward and encourage the man to be aware of and acknowledge his female properties. Similarly, the woman must recognize that that she possesses male properties, and must be aware of them and link up to them. There is no area in life in which this ability is so important as in people's sexuality.

Here is the explanation: the male lover is supposed to reveal the soft, submissive, passive and yielding side of his nature. The woman, in turn, is encouraged to reveal the strong, domineering, motivating and vigorous side of her nature.

This does not mean that the man must relinquish his masculinity altogether or that the woman must relinquish her femininity altogether. Far from it. What this means is that both of them must broaden their nature in order to include the other end of the spectrum. Successful sexual union is experienced as the perfect union of male and female, and so lovers must be tuned in and linked to both their male and their female properties.

The two complementary elements of male and female are represented by the two gods – the god Shiva and his wife, the goddess Shakti. The universe was created from the original union of Shiva and Shakti. According to the Hindu belief, Shiva is considered to be the fertilizing force and is represented by a phallus, the male sex organ, or lingam. Conversely, the goddess Shakti is symbolized by the female sex organ, or yoni. Accordingly, the two gods possess a rich symbolism and sexual significance.

The Taoists had a similar belief. They believed that the world was created from the balanced relations between male and female, which are known in Tao as yang and yin. According to the Tao wisdom, the sexual union between a man and a woman is symbolized by the union between yang and yin, or between heaven and earth.

The man and the woman each possess both yang and yin properties, and it is only a question of which aspect is the dominant one – a question that determines whether a person is a man or a woman. The meeting between yin and yang creates the sexual energy, "o ching," which is expressed in the life force.

Yin and yang are represented by a circle that is divided into two parts. A curved line between the two parts separates the yin, which is black, from the yang, which is white. In the center of each part, there is a dot in the other color, symbolizing the fact that the two can never be separated from each other.

8

During sex, sexual energy moves in the human body, and it is possible to feel and use its movement in a positive and beneficial way. In other words, the energy increases during the sexual arousal stage and can be channeled in the desired direction.

9

The Indian Tantra texts speak about the existence of seven energy centers in the human body. These centers are known as chakras, and the body's energy is stored in them. The chakras are represented as lotus flowers, and each petal is supposed to represent the blooming of a particular quality or area in the person's life. Each of the chakras belongs to an Indian god who also characterizes it. Furthermore, there are several symbolic animals, sounds, colors and gemstones that are associated with it and affect it, and a particular psychological or spiritual activity is attributed to each one.

By opening and balancing the chakras, the learning process of tantric sex and its application may be reinforced. The opening and balancing of the chakras may enable us not only to practice the art of Tantra more efficiently, but also to effect a change in our entire way of life.

Therefore, it is worthwhile going to a skilled therapist (or healer) who specializes in opening and balancing chakras, or to broaden our knowledge of the subject. It is also possible to help open and balance the chakras by ourselves. A relatively good and safe way is by placing suitable gemstones on the chakras. (A more detailed explanation appears later on in the book.)

10

In conclusion, study the principles of Tantra and follow them. You may well discover that tantric sex is one of the best things you've ever done. It may turn out to be beneficial to you in an indescribable way. However, even if it does not make such an enormous and drastic change in your life, it can be a tremendous pleasure!

Chapter 3

Chakras

The seven energy centers

There are seven principal chakras that are located along the vertical line of the body – from the base of the spine to the crown of the head. Below are the seven energy centers, from the base upward:

1
The base chakra –
Muladhara

This chakra is known as the "base" or "root" chakra. It is located at the base of the spine, between the anus and the genitals, in an area called the perineum.

This chakra, which oversees our instincts, is an extremely powerful source of passion and is associated with the sensation of life and with survival. Its colors are red and black, and the symbol that represents it is a circle surrounded by four lotus leaves with a square inside it. Sometimes, the square is colored yellow-gold.

The chakra is identified with the element of earth, the sense of smell, the energy of vitality and the coccyx nerve plexus. The age at which the chakra develops extends from birth to three to five years.

The base chakra, which is the first chakra, is associated with the spine and the skeleton, the teeth and the nails, and the body's excretory organs – the anus, rectum and intestines, the reproductive organs and those of physical continuity, the prostate and the gonads, as well as the blood and the building of cells. The hormonal glands that are associated with it are the sex and the adrenal glands.

The base chakra is considered to be the one that links us to the material world. Its action enables high energies to pass into the person's physical layers, and the stabilizing energy of the earth to be transmitted to the person's energetic bodies. As its name implies, being the "base" or "root" is in fact its action: it forms the basis of the action of the other chakras and the basis of the person's existence and development.

Tantric Sex

Through the root chakra, we feel the roots deep in the earth, from which we receive vital force, nutrition and stability. The function of the base chakra is to give us a feeling of confidence and stability, which is what people need for developing. When a person has roots that go deep into the earth, and a feeling of a solid, stable and secure base, he can also develop on the mental and spiritual layers in a healthy and stable manner.

The base chakra arouses the person's basic survival instinct: the need to work in order to attain stability and to find sufficient healthful food, as well as the need for shelter and continuity. It is also the chakra that activates the sexual instincts. (While it activates them, the awareness of the sexual instincts is attributed to the second chakra, the sex chakra. The sexuality that is attributed to the first chakra is more in the sense of survival and continuity, that is, the procreation of the next generation.)

The need to safeguard oneself against danger – the person's most basic and primal need – originates in the action of this chakra. This gives rise to the instincts we employ for defending ourselves and for preserving our physical and mental wellbeing, as well as the readiness to fight to obtain and provide ourselves with basic commodities such as food and shelter. The first chakra also represents the positive aspect of fear – the one that prevents us from getting into a situation that is liable to endanger us, such as the fear that prevents us from putting our hands in fire or from jumping into deep water.

The key words that represent the action of the chakra are rootedness, stability, acceptance, self-preservation, survival and understanding, and physical will power for existence and survival.

Heightening Sexual Pleasure

When there is an imbalance in the functioning of the chakra, the person is liable to be fraught with fears such as a lack of connection to the ground, dependence on other people's opinions, an unhealthy attitude toward money – over-accumulation of money and devoting too much thought to the material aspects of life – or, on the other hand, a complete and unhealthy disdain of the material facet of life.

Furthermore, he could manifest a "rebellion" of his basic existential instincts, and this would reveal itself in exaggerated risk-taking. On the physical layer, the imbalance may manifest itself in problems such as constipation, hemorrhoids, fatigue, apathy, listlessness, blood ailments, problems and tension in the spine, joints and bones, and tissue and skin problems.

The rishis, the sages of India, attributed the sound "lam" to the base chakra as a means of balancing it. The crystals and minerals that are used to balance the chakra are agate, ruby, onyx, hematite, red jasper, bloodstone, red coral, cuprite, garnet, jet, rhodochrosite, spinel, smoky quartz, alexandrite and black tourmaline. Most of the stones are dark to black and red stones, that is, stones that "respond" to the colors of the chakra.

2
The sex chakra – Svadhisthana

The second chakra, known as the "navel chakra" or the "sex chakra," is located in the genital region, on the pelvis, between the pubic bones. This chakra controls our sexuality. Its importance to Tantra is enormous, but in order to make the person whole (this wholeness is also expressed in his spiritual ability and the spiritual elation that is derived from Tantra), all of the chakras must be open and balanced.

As regards Tantra, the importance of the sex chakra lies more in our perception of sexuality in general, and of our own sexuality in particular. The color of the sex chakra is generally orange, but it can also be yellow-orange. The symbol of the chakra is a circle surrounded by five lotus petals. Sometimes, the circle contains the shape of a half-crescent in a silvery-gray color, and sometimes the chakra is represented as a white crescent. The element that is identified with it is water – the element that represents movement and emotions. The sense associated with it is taste, and the energy associated with it is creative energy. This chakra controls the pelvic nerve plexus, and the time range of its development is between the ages of three and eight. The organs associated with the second chakra are the pelvis, the lymphatic system, the kidneys, the bladder, the muscles, the sex organs, and all of the bodily fluids – blood, lymph, digestive juices and semen. The glands that are associated with it are the ovaries, the testicles, the prostate and the lymphatic system.

Heightening Sexual Pleasure

The second chakra is the center of the sexual and creative energies as well as of the primal non-differentiated emotions. It symbolizes our self-perception as individuals, together with the ability to understand the difference and the uniqueness of the Other and the changes and transformations that occur in life.

The energies of the second chakra draw their power from the energies of the base chakra, which supplies it with a basis and stability. Therefore, the equilibrium of the second chakra actually depends on the equilibrium of the first. This is very important to tantric training, because when the properties of stability, basis and confidence – which stem from the balanced state of the first chakra – are absent, the person is liable to suffer from a lack of confidence and self-doubt regarding his abilities. This can sometimes be reflected in the sexual realm as a lack of sexual confidence.

The opening and balancing of the sex chakra is also important for us to be able to sense and feel the Other, the second person – an ability without which good and genuine sex cannot bloom and flourish. When the chakra is balanced, we are considerate of the feelings of the Other and include them in our thoughts, according to our relationship with him. When both chakras are balanced, we have the confidence and ability to experience the other person as separate from us, but at the same time, as a part of us. This ability is fundamental to the practice of Tantra. In this way, we can display sensitivity, empathy and consideration, but at the same time also be objective and independent. As stated above, this chakra is the center of sexuality, that is, the center of sexual enjoyment as well as the center of sexual desire and fertility.

As we said previously, the base chakra is responsible for

the sexual instincts, the ones that cause us to perpetuate ourselves via reproduction. The sex chakra, however, is responsible for the broader meaning of sexuality, and it relates directly to the sexual act itself – that is, the way in which we perceive our sexuality, our ability to accept our gender with love, and the way in which we accept and see ourselves as a woman or a man. The sex chakra controls sexual awareness, the awareness of sex in general, sexual choice, and the feelings and associations regarding sex.

We can therefore understand why balancing and opening this chakra are important for tantric practice; this energy center stores our sexual patterns as well as other patterns that are instilled in us by society. It absorbs sexual norms as well as the attitude toward sex that is prevalent in our surroundings when we are young children. These norms can reflect a natural, normal, accepting and appreciative attitude toward sexuality – but conversely, they can reflect something that creates a serious barrier that must be eliminated when we begin our tantric training: feelings of "forbidden," "dirty," "sinful" and so on. In the same way, the beliefs regarding "the man's role" and "the woman's role" both in the relationship and in bed are stored in this chakra. When we examine the functions of the sex chakra, we can clearly see the link between impulsiveness and creativity, and between sexuality and creation.

Just as this chakra is responsible for the higher sexual functions, so it is responsible for the ability to create, to produce and to give birth – physically, emotionally and artistically. It is responsible for the ability to embrace change and development, seek adventure and innovation, display curiosity and the desire to explore the unknown, and accept change positively, as well as not to cling to what exists at any price.

Heightening Sexual Pleasure

It is also the chakra that helps us put things into practice, externalize things that are inside us, activate our potential and aspire to realize it, thereby expressing our uniqueness and our unique talents (without being afraid of the reactions of our surroundings). It causes us to be responsible for and in control of our power without relinquishing it or wasting it on others.

This chakra enables us to be a part of the whole, a part of society and the community while maintaining the integrity of our own uniqueness without feeling the need to "smooth over" or change our opinions and beliefs because they ostensibly do not tally with those of our surroundings. This means self-acceptance and belief in oneself and in one's inner strength as well as an absence of fear of social rejection as a result of maintaining one's individuality and uniqueness.

Moreover, the balanced state of the chakra is reflected in uniqueness and individuality that are dedicated to helping nurture society, family and the environment. The person feels that he is an active partner in his family or in his community, and functions in a positive and stable manner in these frameworks. To a certain extent, this is one of the essential properties of Tantra – the ability to be an individual but also the ability for full engagement.

This ability to be one and to be a part without forgoing one's sense of self gives rise to one of the other functions of the chakra – the ability to be honest. Honesty is one of the essential cornerstones for the practice of Tantra and for true enjoyment of sex. If we are unable to be honest in a relationship both in and out of bed, it will not be a genuine relationship, and it will not be genuine sexual enjoyment. Honesty is not just honesty with the other person, but also honesty with oneself.

Tantric Sex

The key words that represent the second chakra are sexuality, creativity, change, a sense of the other, honesty, sensitivity, inner strength and confidence.

If the sex chakra is in a state of imbalance or blockage, the person is liable to be uncaring toward others, excessively self-centered or very dependent. An imbalance in the chakra is liable to affect sexual function and outlook significantly. The person is liable to have an unhealthy attitude toward sex, to feel that sex is "polluted," "impure," "forbidden," and so on. Furthermore, he is liable to be afraid of touching himself and giving himself pleasure, to feel a lack of sexual confidence (which causes sexual dysfunction and sometimes even the fear of establishing deep ties with members of the opposite sex), and to suffer from impotence or a lack of sexual desire or passion. On the other hand, the person is liable to get into a pattern of having sex indiscriminately, without really wanting to or enjoying it; sometimes he even becomes obsessed with sex. Similarly, various addictions can also be symptoms of an unbalanced sex chakra.

From the physical point of view, an imbalance in the sex chakra may be expressed in physical problems such as muscle cramps, allergies, physical exhaustion, constipation, sexual imbalance and a lack of sexual desire, sterility, inhibitions and repressed emotions, and a lack of creativity. The rishis consider the sound "vam" to be the sound that is associated with balancing the chakra. The gemstones and crystals that are used to balance the chakra are mainly orange, golden and yellow-orange in color, and include amber, citrine, topaz, moonstone, fire agate, orange spinel and fire opal.

3
The solar plexus chakra - Manipuraka

This chakra is also known by the names "Manipura," "solar plexus chakra" or "navel chakra." Some people mark its location in the middle of the stomach, directly below the navel, while others claim that it is located below the diaphragm, that is, from the sternum to above the navel.

The solar plexus chakra oversees our personal strength and is identified with strength, vitality and ambition. The color that represents it is yellow, and it is symbolized by a circle surrounded by ten lotus petals containing a triangle (usually red), and sometimes only by a red triangle. This chakra is associated with the element of fire and the sense of sight. The energy that represents it is inner strength. It is associated with the solar plexus nerve plexus, and the time range of its development is between the ages of eight and twelve.

The organs that are associated with the third chakra are the respiratory system and the diaphragm, the digestive system, the stomach, the pancreas, the liver, the spleen, the gallbladder, the small intestine, the extra-renal glands, the lower back and the sympathetic nervous system. The pancreas and the adrenal gland are the hormonal glands for which it is responsible.

This chakra is the center of the individual's personal strength. Through its action, we create an active tie with other people and with the physical world. It is responsible for our personal development and our ability to broadcast our emotions to the world, to affect our surroundings and to direct our inner strength into voluntary activities. It also represents our ego and the practical facet of our intellect.

The state of this chakra affects the way in which we connect to the world and interpret it. It is the center of personal strength, will, ego and self-realization. Its importance in Tantra is expressed mainly in the ability to establish relationships with other people – balanced and long-term relationships. These abilities are vital for the true and correct practice of Tantra. This approach is very important with regard to the emotional layer, as it is with regard to the ability to be aware of our wishes and of the things we like or do not like (a very important ability when having sex).

In a more general sense, the chakra is responsible for the desire for recognition and social status, for structural identity in society, a desire and aspiration for power, for achievement, for accomplishing goals and realizing ambitions, and for adopting social patterns.

Since it is the chakra that represents the ego, it is also linked to the ability to construct a rational attitude and to express an opinion about life, to be able to make decisions, and to form and consolidate personal opinions. The solar plexus chakra is characterized by logic, rationality and intelligence, since these are in fact a continuation of the process of individualization that occurs in the second chakra.

The logic that stems from the third chakra helps us find our direction in life and express our uniqueness while finding our place and status in society. Manipuraka is also the center that enables us to assimilate the knowledge and experience required for forming our personality. Through this chakra, we feel the vibrations and energies of the people around us and operate accordingly. Manipuraka has great importance from the spiritual point of view, since it channels the desires and wishes that are directed to it from the lower chakras for spiritual development. In other words, it serves as a transit station between the lower chakras and the upper chakras. By means of this action, therefore, it is possible to use the primal, basic creative energy for spiritual activity.

In fact, the spiritual role of the chakra is to help us realize our calling in the material world, that is, to play our life role as best we can, using our abilities and our talents, and to walk along the path of our personal fate in the material world in order to achieve self-realization in all the layers.

When the lower chakras (the base and sex chakras) are open and balanced, emotions, passions and expectations serve as material for the development of the third chakra as well as for understanding the events that occur in our lives. (This understanding and these abilities will become pure spirituality only when they merge into the energetic current of the heart and third eye chakras.)

When the third chakra is open, we can receive the sunlight and allow it to sparkle inside us and to illuminate what is outside of us. There is a feeling of joy, cheerfulness, happiness and contentment, abundance and intellectual comprehension.

We broadcast all of these to the world and gain experience in accordance with what we broadcast.

An imbalance in this chakra is liable to create a feeling of general imbalance, sadness, constant preoccupation with material existence and the lower layers of existence, egoism, a powerful desire to control one's internal and external world, an unbalanced ego, a fierce need for status and honor (sometimes even to the detriment of other people in the quest to accomplish personal goals), manipulative behavior, domineering behavior, arrogance, abuse of power, a need to amass more and more power, excessive competitiveness and ambitiousness, a constant restlessness, a lack of fulfillment, a feeling of worthlessness, constant self-judgment according to material or social criteria, over-activity, an inability to relax, the repression of emotions or ignoring them, the rejection of the emotional world in favor of the material world (sometimes to the point that the emotions are repressed but burst out in a dangerous way), feelings of anger and bitterness, sometimes camouflaged as indifference or pretence, outbursts of rage or attacks of depression, feelings of detachment from other people, ties based solely on personal interests, the inability to create genuine ties of closeness and friendship, fear of the inner strength, exhaustion, a feeling of being rejected by one's surroundings, a lack of courage, a feeling that the world is filled with insurmountable obstacles, a need for the constant approval of one's surroundings, the repression of emotions, a lack of assertiveness, an inability to stand up for one's opinions, dependence, various fears, agitation, and the inability to face challenges.

On the physical layer, an imbalance in this chakra is liable to be reflected in problems of mental and nervous exhaustion, gallstones, diabetes, digestive problems, ulcers, allergies and cardiac problems.

The key words that describe this chakra are self-knowledge, logic, cause, action, integration, and personal strength.

The Indian rishis considered the sound "ram" to address the chakra. The stones and crystals that are suitable for balancing it are mainly yellow and golden stones that include citrine, amber, tiger-eye, peridot, yellow tourmaline and golden topaz.

4
The heart chakra –
Anahata

The fourth chakra is also called the "heart chakra." It is located parallel to the line of the heart, but in the middle. This chakra is thought to oversee our love lives. Anahata is usually symbolized by a circle surrounded by 12 lotus petals containing a six-pointed star that is sometimes painted blue. The colors that indicate the chakra are green and pink.

The heart chakra is identified with the element of air and with the sense of touch. The energy it represents is harmony. The time range of its development is between the ages of 13 and 15. The organs associated with it are the heart, the circulatory system, the lungs, the immune system, the thymus gland, the upper back, the skin and the hands; the hormonal gland it influences is the thymus gland.

Anahata is the chakra that links the three lower chakras with the three upper chakras, so its balance is vital for the balance of all the chakras.

It serves as the center of caring about the Other, of giving, of love and devotion, and of the ability to feel and sense the other person, both emotionally and physically. Its importance in the practice of Tantra is enormous. Through it, the person senses the one he loves, and, by means of this connection, can activate his ability to link up to the entire universe and to the divine power – an ability that is the most sublime gift of Tantra.

Sights, sounds and words are translated into emotion in

the heart chakra. Because of it, we aspire to love and are able to love, to give and receive love without self-interest or ego, thereby opening ourselves to divine love. This chakra inspires in us the aspiration for harmony and unity in all layers. In Tantra, this unity is achieved by arousing the love for one's partner, thereby in fact sparking the ability to open up to celestial love and to faith (an ability that stems from the fifth center, the "throat chakra).

Just as the solar plexus chakra is responsible for self-esteem, so the heart chakra is responsible for self-love. How is it possible to love another person truly – without complexes, dependence or other by-products that are sometimes mistakenly thought to be "love" – without self-love?

Complete self-love is essential for love of the Other. In order to attain the ability to link up to the universal force – which is the sublime and pure goal of Tantra – beyond sexual pleasure alone, we must learn to love ourselves and the Other and to accept ourselves and the Other. This chakra is the one that teaches us to forgive, excuse, be compassionate, give of ourselves, love with non-judgmental understanding and feel empathy toward another person.

The basic emotions are created and formed in the sex chakra and activated in relation to the "I" in the solar plexus chakra and the heart chakra to become conscious emotions that develop into the ability to feel other people and to be less self-centered. The opening of the heart causes the person to allow himself to be sensitive, to expose his inner side and to be soft and loving. This softness is expressed in physical contact (but not only in physical contact) and it is also reflected in all of the person's interactions with others, and of course with himself.

Tantric Sex

The opening of the heart affords us the strength to be sensitive and without protective layers and armor in relationships. Together with being responsible for empathy and the ability to identify with others, the heart chakra is also responsible for the vital aspect of this ability – the ability to be ourselves. We must not reach a point of such profound identification with someone else that we lose our sense of self or take on someone else's pain. It also enables us to detach ourselves and see things objectively so that we can really and truly help.

For this reason, the key words that represent the heart chakra are love, harmony, devotion, softness, compassion, emotion and balance.

When the heart chakra is not balanced, or is blocked, the person finds it difficult to give or receive love. His abilities to give and receive are deficient or unbalanced in some way. He is liable to give and give until he reaches the point of exhaustion, because he is not linked to the true center of love. He is liable to be embarrassed about showing affection, to interpret softness and affection as weakness, to feel that he is not worthy of love and therefore cannot give it, either, or to be incapable of allowing himself to expose his emotions.

Furthermore, the person may be very sensitive and vulnerable and afraid to express his feelings. He is liable to create a protective covering, to be dependent on the approval and love of others, to be spineless and lacking in self-confidence, to find it difficult to establish a real and open relationship with other people, and to fear abandonment, rejection and the loss of love.

Sometimes the person is liable to be cold and indifferent, with a "heart of stone," depressed, tense, nervous, and in extreme cases, even evil. He is liable to lack the ability to forgive, and he may be irascible, jealous and stingy – physically or emotionally. Of course, these emotional symptoms do not all appear in one person; their occurrence depends on the type of imbalance that exists in the person's heart chakra.

On the physical layer, the imbalance of the heart chakra is liable to be reflected in the following ways: cardiac pains, heart attacks, hypertension, respiratory difficulties, tension, insomnia, fatigue, and various states of emotional imbalance.

The rishis of India chose the sound "yam" as the sound that addresses the chakra. The crystals and stones that affect the chakra and help balance it are mainly green and pink in color, and include rose quartz, aventurine, chrysocolla, emerald, jade, chrysoprase, dioptase, malachite, rhodonite and so on.

5
The throat chakra – Vishudda

Vishudda, or Vishadha, is also known as the "throat chakra" because it is located in the region of the throat between the bones of the clavicle. Vishudda is the chakra that oversees everything to do with communication, so it belongs to the fields of speech, expression and creativity.

The colors that represent it are blue, light blue and turquoise. It is usually represented as a white circle or as a circle surrounded by 16 lotus petals with another circle inside it, or a circle with a triangle in it. The sense for which it is responsible is hearing. The energy it represents is Vishudda, which is the energy of self-expression. The time range of its development is between the ages of 15 and 21. The organs associated with it are the throat, the neck, the vocal cords and the vocal organs, the thyroid gland, the parathyroid glands, the jaw, the top part of the lungs, the nerves, the ears, the muscles and the arms. The glands for which it is responsible are the thyroid and the parathyroid glands.

Vishudda, the fifth chakra, is the center of communication, inspiration and human expression. It is responsible for all facets of communication – self-communication, communication with the Other, and communication with the universal force.

The fifth chakra connects thought and the ability to express the thought (using any form of expression). Vishudda is also responsible for our self-image, and serves as a bridge between our thoughts, emotions, urges and reactions, while expressing the entire contents of the other chakras outwardly to the world, in its capacity of the center of expression.

Through the fifth chakra, we express our feelings, joy, sadness, vitality and love consciously, actively and clearly. There is a powerful and unique bond between the throat chakra – which is responsible for inspiration – and the sex chakra, which is responsible for creativity. It is the one that raises creativity to the level of artistic expression. The more open and balanced Vishudda is, the more the person can know and be aware of what is going on inside him. He can distinguish the urges, needs and emotions that are at work in him, and sort themselves out for himself objectively. He decides what to project outward and what to keep to himself. He makes the decision to get rid of what is not of use to him.

The fifth chakra is also the center that is responsible for our ability to listen – the other side of the ability of expression. Listening creates tranquillity, calmness and confidence in the person, and unites the ability to define the inner world with the ability to discern truly and clearly what is happening in the external world.

When the chakra is open and balanced, the person has self-confidence and a positive and stable self-image. Even if various incidents occur or he is subjected to negative criticism, the person knows that he has self-worth, and is therefore not afraid of mistakes and failure. He knows that come what may, he will always be himself. He feels confidence and faith in divine guidance, and he possesses the will to realize his cosmic calling and to express himself in the layers beyond the material and existential layer.

The imagination also falls under the aegis of this chakra,

as does the sense of responsibility: (1) responsibility toward oneself – responsibility for one's development, for one's personal life, for the body's health and nutrition; and (2) responsibility toward others and their good. This chakra also directs us to maintain law and order, and, on the highest level, to aspire to universal truth; conscience, justice, truth, honesty, the aspiration for peace – these qualities are the fruit of the activity of the fifth chakra.

The key words for Vishudda are communication, expression, responsibility, honesty, will power, self-esteem, universal truth, faith.

When Vishudda is open and balanced, the person can express his feelings, thoughts, opinions and his inner knowledge clearly, fearlessly and freely. He feels sure of himself and is not afraid to expose his strengths and weaknesses to others. He has a correct and positive self-image, is responsible, possesses an inner honesty, aspires to peace and has faith. Furthermore, he has a good listening ability (as well as a good ability to express himself) and a certain stability in his beliefs and opinions. As a result of this stability, he is prepared to listen to new and different opinions.

He has the ability to set limits when necessary and to be flexible when appropriate, and he feels free, non-reliant and independent of others. He is decisive and aware of himself, and recognizes his weaknesses just as he recognizes his abilities and qualities. In such a person, harmony reigns between reason and emotion. He is free from prejudices and enjoys good control over his thoughts, and this enables him to enter meditative states (a very important ability for Tantra, as we will see later on) and communicate with the "upper I."

In contrast, when the throat chakra is not open or balanced, there might be difficulties in self-expression and problems in communication (between the person himself and his body) as a result of his not knowing how to "listen" to his body and to his emotions and desires. There could be communication problems between him and other people as well.

A breach between thought and emotion may occur, as may conflicts between emotion and reason. The person could suffer from low self-esteem, a lack of confidence, constant self-criticism, a fear of expressing opinions and beliefs, guilt feelings, speech problems – both in speech itself, such as stammering, and in the ability to transfer his thought to the verbal level clearly and fluently. Sometimes, he is afraid of "betraying" weaknesses and pretends to be strong at any price. Furthermore, a blockage in this energetic center may also be reflected in a lack of creativity and a lack of imagination.

Sometimes a tendency toward garrulousness, gossiping, emotional outbursts (because emotions are repressed) and bitterness may appear – or, conversely, apathy and indifference. The person is liable to be shy, uninvolved, uncomfortable in company and lacking in confidence in his personal intuition. He may find it difficult to understand what is beyond physical reality, and he may fear the future.

An imbalance in Vishudda, from the physical point of view, is liable to manifest itself in the following things: speech problems, breathing problems, headaches, pains in the neck, shoulders and nape, problems and inflammations in the throat, problems with the vocal cords, and inflammations, infections and problems in the ears.

The Indian rishis chose the sound "yam" as the sound

that addresses the fifth chakra. The crystals and minerals that are used to balance and open the chakra are mainly shades of blue, light blue and turquoise, and include sapphire, turquoise, sodalite, blue lace agate, lapis lazuli, chrysocolla, blue quartz, blue tourmaline, aquamarine, and so on.

6
The third eye chakra –
Ajna

Ajna is known as the "third eye chakra," and it is located between the eyebrows. Ajna oversees our intellect and is associated with intuition, perception and imagination.

The colors that represent it are indigo and purple. It is symbolized by a sky-blue circle surrounded on both sides by large lotus petals, and inside it is a drawing of two feet. Sometimes it is also symbolized by an inverted white triangle. The element that is identified with it is radium, and the sense associated with it is the intuition (the "sixth sense"), as well as all the senses in their most subtle, extrasensory, form. The energy that represents it is the intuition.

The organs for which it is responsible are the brain and its various components, the central nervous system, the face, eyes, ears, nose and sinuses. The glands that are associated with it are the pituitary and the pineal glands.

The third eye chakra is said to be "the daughter of the father Shiva." Some of the Tantra exponents compare this chakra to the feeling a person is likely to experience when he reaches the summit of a high mountain after an exhausting climb. The meaning of the name "Ajna" in Sanskrit is "control center." It is exactly like its name – the third eye is responsible for conscious perception, and oversees the various mental abilities, the memory, will power and knowledge.

It links us to our subconscious, to the intuition, to the ability to understand cosmic insights and receive nonverbal messages. In addition, it is responsible for the balance between the two hemispheres of the brain, the right and the left – between intuition, emotion and mysticism on the one hand and reason and logic on the other. Moreover, it is responsible for the person's physical balance, for the ability to concentrate, for peace of mind and for wisdom.

Ajna arouses in us the desire for a feeling of wholeness, the desire to feel perfect harmony with the universe – which sometimes happens at the higher levels of the practice of Tantra. It is not open in many people, so very few experience such a feeling, and few ask questions like "Who am I?" "What is my place in the universe?" "What is beyond the physical universe?" Most people perceive the existing reality as the only reality.

When the chakra is opened (sometimes as a result of tantric training), the person experiences a desire to feel this harmony with the universe, initially with himself.

At first, various questions arise, as well as a desire for self-perfection, for honesty to oneself, for belief in what man does, and a feeling that there are lofty forces at work in the universe, of which man is part. The person begins to be aware of his soul, and may even undergo some crisis (whose results may well be positive), in which he feels that "normal" life – accumulating assets, economic security, work, status and so on – is not fulfilling. This crisis may lead him to a search for himself and for the development of awareness. He begins to desire equilibrium and harmony between body, intellect, emotions, soul and spirit.

It is worthwhile mentioning that Ajna plays a significant role in creation; it links the person to inspiration and innovation.

As we stated above, the meaning of the name of the

chakra is "control center." It controls the nervous system, and when it is balanced and open, it enables us to oversee and take control of our lives. When it is open, we can see how we ourselves create our reality, and how our thoughts and beliefs are embodied and manifested in a physical and practical way. The person can look inside his set of beliefs and patterns and eliminate what does not support him, as well as the things to which he adhered because of various social norms, but do not in fact contain any truth.

The chakra is also responsible for our intuitive ability, for extrasensory perception and for the ability to use the extrasensory senses. Sometimes its opening goes hand in hand with the development of various extrasensory abilities such as premonitions, telepathy and so on.

The key words that describe the action of the chakra are existential awareness, inspiration, spirituality, command and perfection.

When the third eye chakra is balanced (even if it is not completely open), the person has a good intellectual ability, a talent for philosophy, research or inventive abilities, clarity of thought, a high sense of morality, a deep sense of social belonging and an ability to establish ties with people easily, the ability to use his imagination and powerful visualization and intuitive powers. He can understand the world and the things that happen in a more profound manner, he can understand how his patterns of belief and thought affect his life, and sometimes even see the "mirrors" of his thoughts and beliefs embodied in the people and life events he encounters.

When the chakra is not balanced, the person is liable to experience his life through intellect and reason only, as a result of a powerful need for order and logic in everything.

What does not seem logical to him is perceived by him to be impossible. To a person who is in a state of extreme imbalance, both intuition and emotions seem illogical. All this is liable to lead to an extremely reduced view of the world as well as to resistance to anything spiritual. On the other hand, in a slightly different state of imbalance, the person may actually possess spiritual understanding, but this understanding is liable to be superficial only, and does not become assimilated in his deeper thoughts and actions, nor does it inspire true commitment to the laws of the universe.

Sometimes, the person is liable to want to use spiritual powers in order to influence people without asking their permission, or for various self-interests. In situations in which the third eye chakra is partially open, but is in a state of imbalance, and the rest of the chakras, especially the lower ones, are not balanced, the person is liable to suffer from a general imbalance, a feeling of floating and a lack of grounding. He is also unable to understand the messages that he picks up via his intuition or distinguish between cosmic truths and things that are figments of his imagination – so much so that he loses touch with reality.

More common is a situation in which the imbalance of Ajna causes a lack of confidence in the universe as well as a lack of in-depth understanding of events and occurrences. This lack of confidence is liable to be reflected in various anxieties, in a lack of tranquillity, in a fear of the future, in indecisiveness, in nervousness, in constantn tension and in cynicism. In addition, problems such as difficulties in comprehension, learning difficulties, a low intellectual capacity and hearing and sight problems are liable to occur when there is a blockage in the chakra. Furthermore, confused and murky thinking, disrupted by irrelevant emotions, may occur. States of imbalance in the chakra are also liable to be reflected in mental exhaustion, depression, numerous unrequited passions, fanaticism, and an inability to relax.

The rishis found the sound "ham – kesham" to be the sound that addresses and affects the third eye chakra. The crystals and minerals that are used for balancing and opening the chakra are mainly indigo and purple in color, and include amethyst, azurite, fluorite, lapidolite and sugelite.

7
The crown chakra – Sahasrara

Sahasrara, also known as the "crown chakra," is located in the crown of the head. The colors that represent it are purple, white, gold and silver, and its symbol is a lotus with a thousand petals. The element that is identified with it is magnetum, and its energy is the energy of thought. The organ associated with the chakra is the cerebrum.

The crown chakra is said to link us with the rest of the world; it is also said to be associated with unity and wisdom. This chakra, as opposed to the others, is different, and does not operate in the same way as they do. It is said that the goddess Shakti resides in it, and the aim of raising the energy from the base chakra upward to the third eye chakra and the crown chakra is supposedly, according to the ancient Sanskrit doctrine, to release Shiva so that he can unite with Shakti.

This is said to make the union between the male and the female principles possible – a union that leads to celestial bliss or illumination – and to give a fortunate person (whose crown chakra is sufficiently developed) the possibility of sex that is a mystical and blissful experience.

This chakra is the center of human perfection. It signifies illumination and linking up to the higher layers of consciousness and spirituality. It unites the energies of all of the lower energetic centers, and links the physical body to the cosmic energy system.

Heightening Sexual Pleasure

Similarly, the crown chakra is responsible for the link to the upper awareness, for the ability to receive divine and cosmic insights, and for the ability to link up to divine knowledge and to the light and universal love.

It is a place in which there is no need for thought, for controlling reality or for activity. It is a place in which there is only pure essence, a place in which it is possible simply to "be." From the action of the crown chakra, we learn to accept ourselves completely – as an energetic part that is inseparable from the entire universe, as a soul that experiences existence in this dimension as well as in other dimensions of the universe.

Here, what we understand intellectually and then intuitively becomes understanding and knowledge. Here there are no questions like "What?" "Why?" "How?" "Where?" but rather only knowledge. The knowledge that comes from the crown chakra is much further-reaching than the knowledge that comes from the third eye chakra because here we are no longer separated from the object of our observation, but rather united with it, and we do not see anything in the universe as separate from us. We understand and know that the Other is actually a part of us and a part of the universe, because of the fact that we are ostensibly the embodiment of energy in a separate body. As a result, devotion, tranquillity, faith and acceptance are stimulated.

When the blockages in the crown chakra are released and it receives energy in a full and perfect manner, all the blockages that remain in the other chakras want to be opened. This is done by using our power of thought and feeling to raise our consciousness to a state in which we can bring the nature of the blockage to the surface and release it by the very fact of understanding it. All of the chakras vibrate at their highest frequencies, and each of them operates as a mirror of the divine essence at its unique level, expressing its full potential.

When the crown chakra is completely aroused, the person begins to project all of the cosmic energies he has absorbed into the cosmos. From being influenced by the energies, he becomes the one who influences them, the force in the universe that works in perfect tandem with the universe. He becomes a "light worker."

The center of the crown, even if it is not usually completely open, may open up during meditation or at high levels of tantric practice. In those moments, it receives divine knowledge that is subsequently processed and comprehended via the rest of the centers and is expressed in thought, speech and deed.

In fact, there is no state of blockage in the crown chakra; it can be more open or less open, and more developed or less developed. The more open it is, the more the person will experience moments in which the difference between external existence and internal existence is blurred and disappears, and he experiences simply "being" in a state of acceptance, which does not involve needs, thoughts, fears and so on.

His consciousness is completely calm, and the person experiences himself as a part of the pure essence that contains everything that exists. The more developed the crown chakra is, the more frequent these moments are, until they become a constant feeling of balance and perfect harmony with the self and with the universe alike.

The path to illumination becomes illumination itself, which can occur in a surprising manner, such as a feeling of awakening to reality. The person feels that he is a channel for the divine light and is prepared to accept this light at any time and in any form. The personal ego no longer functions as an inhibiting factor, but rather serves as a tool for carrying out God's wishes and is guided by the soul. There is no more resistance or conflict, just acceptance and resignation. The person translates the Creator's intention into deed, speech and thought, and realizes it in the physical world.

The person can accept the answers from the universe via his soul – which is a part of him. He does not feel a need "to do", but rather does; he does not feel embarrassed or uncomfortable, accepts himself in his entirety, and knows how to see everything in the universe as a significant sign. He recognizes emotions such as fear, anger, criticism and sadness as tools for additional development, for additional understanding, and knows how to retreat deep inside himself in order to become acquainted with the source of these emotions and resolve them. He does not attribute them to the "outside," but understands that they come from within him, whether as a mirror or as a need for an experience of that kind in order to learn.

From here, he continues his spiritual development and experiences life as a fascinating game. He understands that he is the one who chose his body, his life, his experiences, and all of those are milestones in the ongoing experience of his soul in the material world. His life is harmonious and happy, and he may well reach a state of illumination.

In contrast, when the crown chakra is usually closed, the person is liable to feel detached and separate from the universe and from the essence. He may feel that his energies are unbalanced and are not in balance with the energies of the universe. He is liable to feel that he lacks a calling; he may be confused, not at one with himself, lacking in basic calmness, full of questions for which he does not know how to get the answers. He may feel bored with life, and a lack of harmony with people, situations, animals and even objects. Moreover, because he lacks a true understanding of the universe, he is liable to experience a fear of death, a feeling that life is futile, a lack of confidence in himself and in the universe, and a lack of wholeness. The person does not see himself as responsible for what happens in his life, and blames "others" or the universe. His ability to develop spiritually is low, and his true potential is not realized.

The sound that the rishis of India attributed to the crown chakra is "om." The crystals and minerals that can be used for opening the chakra are diamond, moldavite, clear quartz, selenite, smithsonite, and pyrite.

The chakras may be open or closed. There are certain activities such as yoga, meditation, dancing, listening to music, and, of course, sex that help accelerate the opening of the chakras, and therefore these activities are highly recommended.

8

Tantric sex enables us to use our body's sexual energy in the correct way. The ultimate goal of good sex is to arouse the extremely powerful energy known as kundalini, which lies dormant at the base of the spine – in the base chakra.

Kundalini is a Sanskrit word that means "curled up." In most cases, the kundalini is described as a sleeping serpent, curled up three and a half times, with its tail in its mouth. The serpent can wreak terrible havoc, or conversely, can invoke tremendous healing powers. The idea is that the moment it is aroused, it rises up via the chakras and has an effect of cleaning and lowering tension with its arousal.

9

Similarly, it is possible to visualize the energy flowing in order to help create energy. As a start, imagine your base chakra and focus your mind on the energy that it creates when it flows upward through your seven chakras. The idea of tantric sex is that your kundalini energy is aroused and rises up through the seven chakras until it finally merges with your partner energy in the upper part of yours heads.

Chapter 4

Preparing the setting, the clothing, and the body for tantric sex

Preparatory steps – the path to perfect enjoyment

1

Rituals constitute an important part of Tantra, and one of them is preparing the setting where the love scene is going to take place. Ritual preparations for sex help create a feeling that sex is really important and special. According to the teachings of Tantra, it is not so important what you do, but rather the time you spend on it. This shows the importance you attribute to lovemaking.

For the tantrists, preparing the setting is a matter of honoring the lover in a sacred, almost festive manner, which, they believed, permits you to yield to the divinity inside you. You may not be ready to go so far in your set of beliefs yet, but there is no doubt that preparing the setting for the event is likely to create the appropriate atmosphere as well as the right mood. This is a practical and useful part of creating intimate ties between two partners.

There are different programs that can be used to create the setting, and different things are suitable and right for different people. For instance, some people find the visual aspects of the room – the lighting and the colors – important. Others find other senses to be dominant – the sense of smell, which is aroused by good and special odors, or the sense of hearing, which is aroused by pleasant and suitable music.

There are no cut and dried rules in this matter, but in most cases, men tend to react better to visual stimulation and women to atmospheric stimulation, such as music and odors.

2

The best way is simply to devote a little time and to give oneself over to preparing the space, preferably with your partner. Use your imagination and make the preparations as slowly and attentively as you can. Make sure that you will not be disturbed, and start with that. Relate to it as a shared experience that will be of great help to both of you, and as a ritual you can enjoy every time before sex. This makes the sexual event unusual, removes it from the ordinary limits and endows it with a special setting. The preparation of your love space is likely to be an erotic event in itself, and may play an important role in igniting the flames of passion or even of rekindling them if the relationship has become somewhat routine.

3
Lighting

Do you like light during sex? Couples sometimes have differences of opinion concerning the amount of lighting during sex. One may prefer darkness while the other likes a little light. In such a case, the two sides should discuss the issue.

In any event, the time devoted to the mutual preparation for blissful sex is really not the time for negotiations or arguments, and there is no doubt that a soft, dim light can be arousing and seductive, and could well suit both of you.

Several lamps around the room undoubtedly create a better atmosphere than a central light fitting, which could be too harsh and powerful, and even cold. The light must not be too bright, but it should imbue the room with a warm and flickering aura.

One of the solutions, of course, is candles. They can produce a dramatic, intimate and magical quality in any room, and create interesting shadows not just in the room in general, but also on the naked skin. This can assist in the arousal of all the senses. Always make sure that the candles are in a safe place where there is no chance that they will endanger the participants by setting fire to fabrics, flowers and so on. Similarly, it is preferable not to place the candles on the floor where they can be kicked or knocked over.

4
Music

A sexual encounter should be an excellent time for two people to listen to music they both like. Listening to the music your partner likes may well be a revealing experience, especially if your musical tastes are different.

Music can get you in the mood and even create an atmosphere. It can also affect your energy level if it is quiet, soothing or stimulating.

Tantric sex supports the need to distance oneself from every prohibition, and music can help in that direction. Dancing can also contain powerful sexual energy, and the tantric writings encourage the couple to dance, together or separately, as a prelude to sex.

5
Fragrance

Some people consider the sense of smell to be the most powerful aphrodisiac available. Accordingly, the use of fragrances you like can help create a suitable atmosphere for sex. A familiar odor can have powerful associations and can help evoke memories of forgotten romantic encounters, while an unfamiliar odor can be a sudden surprise and cause a sensual arousal.

Use an essential oil burner to spread a fragrance throughout the room, or mix a few drops of choice aromatic oil in a plant spray (that has not contained any chemicals!) and spray the room with the mixture.

6
Purification ceremony

Taking a shower or a bath together and washing each other before sex can be an enjoyable and important part of foreplay.

To be clean and fragrant before making love is always a good idea, since it permits the pleasure of the natural odors of the newly-washed body to arouse the senses.

However, when the two members of the couple wash each other, the whole thing takes on a completely different meaning. It is also a symbolic act, which shows very powerfully how all the negative feelings and tensions are washed away.

7
Food and drink

Going to dinner together is something that many couples enjoy, and it can be a significant part of your relationship. Eating and drinking in themselves are high-level sensual activities, and they can be an enjoyable prelude to sex. Food and drink can have excellent properties that can serve to intensify sexual power.

It is important to stress that it is not a good idea to eat too much. If you finish the meal with a feeling of fullness and satiation, it is liable not to arouse sexual potency and activity, and may even put you to sleep. Therefore, be careful, and eat light meals that contain nutritious and fresh food that are both nourishing and healthful for body and mind. Some couples enjoy taking food and drink to bed, and many of us will agree that breakfast in bed together can be a very sexy thing, both before and after sex.

Eating in bed can be a tremendous pleasure (if we can completely ignore the idea of crumbs of toast in the bed and other types of mess, forget about the urge to tidy and clean up, and simply get on with the pleasure itself!). This kind of pleasure is certainly what the tantrists believe that sex should be!

8

Very few Indian, Chinese or Japanese pictures depict lovers who are completely naked. This stresses how erotic a partially clothed lover is considered to be.

The tantrists believe that dressing provocatively for your lover is acceptable and even highly recommended.

They support adorning the face and body with makeup, body paint and jewelry. They also have no problem with the lovers exchanging clothing – something that for some reason shocks many people in our modern culture. The tantrists rule that anything that can make sex more pleasurable, unusual and special is a good idea and adds vitality and interest to the wonderful activity.

Sex while partially clothed allows the body to rub against fabric, which can be very erotic. Experiment with the sensations of different fabrics – silk sheets, for instance, or fur covers.

Anything that adds interest and excitement to sex can increase the pleasure, and you can allow yourselves to be as daring and imaginative as you want.

Remember that according to the writings of the Tantra masters, nothing is forbidden. Absolutely nothing (except, of course, sex that is not consensual and fully desired by both parties, which is despicable and wretched in the extreme and is not considered by the Tantra sages to be sex at all); if it is pleasurable, it's fine, recommended and even worth trying. So don't hold back – go for it and enjoy yourselves...

9

The body is considered to be a temple, the place where matter and spirit meet. For that reason, the tantrists had tremendous respect for their bodies, and in order to prepare them for performing tantric sex, they groomed them and lavished a great deal of attention on them. They believed in improving the levels of physical fitness, since this rewards us with a healthy and pliant body.

It is very important to be aware of the body and its potential, since by doing so, we will have a better and more varied ability to achieve sexual happiness. This is necessary not only for performing actions that lead to physical pleasure, but also for the inherent gift that we can give another person.

10
Yoga

Yoga is an important preparation in the tantric faith. The meaning of the Indian word yoga is "union" or "joining," which relates to the joining of the individual to the deepest layers of consciousness. Yoga is the development of physical stability and positions that not only train the body and strengthen the muscles, but also strengthen the inner organs. In fact, yoga strengthens the entire body both inside and outside.

Heightening Sexual Pleasure

As a result, the highest goal of yoga is to direct the awareness and the energy flow inward, which enables you to experience your body from the inside. This releases both physical and mental tension.

Yoga brings about an awareness of the body, which is one of the most basic requirements for marvelous sex, so it is perhaps the best preparation for tantric sex. Yoga promotes all three of the most important elements of physical fitness: flexibility, endurance and strength. All these are required as a preparation for the best love positions, particularly those that are especially advanced or complex. Yoga also promotes peace of mind, so that the person can remain concentrated and lucid. Tantric practice requires a clear and focused mind all the time.

If yoga is new to you, the best thing may be to join a yoga class in which you can learn and practice all the positions. And then, when you are sure of how to assume the positions by yourself, you will also be able to practice yoga at home or with a friend.

You may want to purchase a book about yoga – preferably a book that includes illustrations or photographs of the positions, as well as detailed instructions as to how to practice them. It is almost certain that in the book you will find explanations about the ways in which each position supports different parts of your body, including certain muscles, organs and bodily functions.

After you have had some practice, you may want to try group yoga again, along with practice at home. An experienced teacher will help ensure that you are performing the positions correctly, and can also teach you about new positions. The best thing is to practice yoga on a daily basis, at least for a few minutes every day. The more frequently you practice these positions, the better you will perform them and the easier they will become.

You may be surprised at how quickly you improve and at your results, which will also reflect your endurance and flexibility. Encouraged by these results, you will quickly go from strength to strength, and in a short time, yoga will become a normal and inseparable part of your lives.

The best time for practicing yoga is in the morning (preferably, it should be your first activity) or early in the evening before eating. It should be done at least two hours after eating. Yoga practice first thing in the morning can make your day different – for the better; while practice in the early evening will help you wind down and relax after a busy day.

There are couples who like to practice yoga together, as part of a group or by themselves at home. This can be enjoyable, and can provide you with a view of the activity of the other person's body. Practicing in the nude can create a strong feeling of unity and intimacy.

11
Breathing

In yoga practice, it is very important to pay attention to your breathing and to make every effort to breathe correctly. We breathe all day, every day, and even so, we so often do not breathe correctly. Yoga can correct this and make you conscious of your breathing. There is a branch of yoga called pranayama in which breathing is considered to be the most important thing.

Being aware of your breathing is very important in good sex (as you will read later on), so anything that can make you understand how to breathe is very valuable. The basic yoga breathing technique is called "the healing breath," and the nature of this breathing constitutes the correct way to breathe.

The best position in which to practice the "healing breath" is lying on your back on the floor or on a hard mattress. Place one hand on your abdomen while you are practicing the breathing. This will enable you to feel the movement of air in and out of your body while you are breathing. Before you begin, exhale all the "stale" breath from your lungs by pushing it out through your nose until your lungs are completely empty.

Afterwards, do the following breathing exercise:

For this exercise, the breath is divided into three parts: inhalation, holding and exhalation. Inhale air until you feel that your abdomen is full, hold your breath to the count of four, exhale it slowly to the count of two, and then let your abdomen contract once more as you empty your lungs.

12
Stress

Nowadays, most people suffer from a great deal of stress. Modern life is very stressful, and tension is liable to accumulate and even to begin to control us. Very few of us succeed in remaining immune to the pressures, and if we are not careful, we are liable to pay a heavy price both physically and mentally.

In everyday life, we are all very busy, and many of us do not have the time to stop and take note of the constant effect that our crazy schedules (which are much too full) have on us. For this reason, we are all liable to become fatigued, tense, nervous, restless and anxious, and one of the first things that suffers from and is jeopardized by the constant tension is our sex lives.

Thus, if we want to experience sexual joy (that tantric sex promises us), the first thing on our list of priorities is to allow ourselves to relax. Taking a break from the insane cauldron of commitments, allowing ourselves to rest a bit, allocating time for rest and relaxation, calming the mind down and finding inner peace – these are not luxuries; they are essential things. Only by doing them will it be possible for us to succeed in opening the inner flow of energy.

Good sex requires both sides to be completely calm, serene and relaxed. Only when you succeed in calming your brain will you be in a suitable frame of mind to achieve a state of acceptance and enjoy every moment of sensual arousal. This state of calm acceptance is totally essential for good sex.

Chapter 5

So when do we start?

Preparing the mind for making love

There are a number of ways in which we can prepare our spirits and minds for the experience of making love. Here are a few of the methods.

1
Relaxation

Effective relaxation is the kind of ability that has to be developed, just like any other acquired and learned ability. (Even though it has always been inherent in us, the feverish pace of life to which we have become accustomed in the Western world has caused many people to forget about it!) It has to be learned and practiced until it is perfected – or until it is as near perfect as possible. In other words, you should practice relaxation until it becomes routine, automatic and second nature to you (such as brushing your teeth in the morning).

Tantric Sex

Relaxation has many advantages. If you are deeply relaxed, your oxygen consumption – which is equivalent to the speed at which your body burns energy – will be drastically reduced. It is worth mentioning that in order to achieve a low level of oxygen consumption, it is generally necessary to sleep for between five and six hours. Accordingly, it is not difficult to understand how healthy and effective profound rest would be. This can be achieved by means of a few minutes of practicing relaxation exercises.

The advantages of relaxation are completely clear. The heart capacity – or the amount of blood that passes through the heart each minute – decreases considerably when you are in a state of deep relaxation. In other words, there is a significant decrease in the heart's workload. For obvious reasons, the heart can never rest completely, but it is clear that overwork at a feverish pace for a long time is liable to be very harmful and even fatal. The heart occasionally needs to reduce its load, and the best way to achieve this is by means of a brief period of deep and effective relaxation.

How exactly you choose to relax depends on you. There are many different ways of relaxing, and different methods suit different people. There are many people who will benefit from engaging in a form of daily exercise such as swimming, a 15-minute walk, or an even more strenuous form of exercise such as riding a bicycle or jogging.

Others find that they can achieve the desired effect by something as simple as listening to music, watching television or reading a gripping book.

In spite of all this, most of us need something a little "stronger" than that. Most of us are far more stressed out than we even imagine, so we have to develop some kind of mechanism that will help us relax. These things are not difficult, but they still have to be learned and practiced (at least for a few minutes each day), and these minutes will make an astounding difference in our lives and state of health.

There are many methods for relaxation. Popular ones included deep breathing exercises, muscle-relaxing exercises, creative visualization, biofeedback, yoga and meditation.

2
Meditation

Meditation is one of the most highly recommended methods of relaxation, especially for people who want to experience the wonders of tantric sex. Meditation has been practiced in the East for hundreds and even thousands of years, and it is central and essential to the life of the yogi, for instance, just as it is to the Tantra practitioner.

There are different forms of meditation that have become religious and cultural experiences – for instance, the meditation of the Sufi Moslems, the Chinese Tao, the Japanese Zen, the Kabbalistic gazing, and so on. Moreover, the medical profession has recently recognized the fact that meditation can be used as an effective form of therapy that releases stress and possesses many well documented and proven advantages – both on the psychological and the physiological levels.

Meditation increases the absorption of oxygen, decreases the heart rate, and lowers body temperature and blood pressure. You do not need "before" and "after" medical tests to notice the immediate and obvious contribution of meditation: time for yourself, with yourself – something that is tremendously valuable in the busy and fast-paced lives we lead.

In our world, there are endless external pressures, demands and obligations as well as "noise" that constantly invades our consciousness ("noise" that comes mainly from the various media, pummeling our brains without our noticing it at all). As a result, the human brain is almost always in a state of constant stimulation, and there is no doubt that it, too, deserves to rest a bit!

Meditation enables you to refresh your inner being, and this can have a dramatic effect of renewal and revival. Meditation means bringing the brain under control in order to free it from various types of distracting and disturbing thoughts. Through meditation, it is possible to achieve a sharp clarity of mind, a clarity that enables you to feel every moment to the full, that is, every moment in which you can feel a powerful feeling of awareness. This creates tremendous advantages in every action you perform in life, and of course also in sex – the reinforcement of the relations between mind and body, a factor that will almost certainly be of tremendous value in your sexual relations.

The next thing will probably surprise you. Meditation, according to the tantric teachings, constitutes one of the most important and sublime tools in the techniques of sex. It does not only relax the brain and leave it free to be calm and focused, but it also reveals the essential person in you and makes your desire to be in contact with your inner I possible.

When you are in touch with your inner I, more direct and focused communication between two people is possible –

in a way that no amount of talking can ever achieve. This encourages a health flow of energy through the human body, a factor that is the essence of tantric sex.

3
Meditation techniques

Like anything else, meditation techniques can be learned. However, it is worth stressing that meditation is not actually focused on doing something; it is more like being in a certain state, a certain state of mind, and therefore it is not possible to compel or force the mind to get into such a state. But it is a most natural state for a person. Therefore, even if initially it is not easy, it is completely feasible for everyone.

If you are prepared for it, if you are in an open, passive and accepting state of mind, ready to accept what may happen unconditionally and fearlessly, entry into this state will occur spontaneously. It can take a long time, or it can happen quickly. It can be something exciting and impressive, and it can also be something very simple, ordinary, calm and wonderful, good and healthy serenity, a few moments of cerebral cleansing. In any case in which meditation occurs, it will be a unique, personal experience, and there is nothing "right" or "wrong" about it. In other words, no two people will have exactly the same experience, so that comparison is irrelevant.

The ideal situation is to practice meditation every day. It will be most effective and beneficial if you practice meditation for ten to twenty minutes, twice a day. However, as a start, if you are not experienced, even a few minutes will suffice. (Count the minutes internally – in other words, don't count. The moment you feel you've had enough, it is a sign that it is enough for the time being.) Gradually you will feel that you can remain in a state of meditation for a longer time. Perform the meditation in a warm, comfortable place in which you can be sure that nobody will disturb you. Turn off the phone, and if there are other people in the house, explain to them what you're doing and ask them to make sure they don't disturb you for some time.

4
Transcendental meditation

A comfortable position is very important in meditation. Generally, meditation is performed sitting up, but it is also possible to do it lying down or standing up. It is worth mentioning that lying down is suitable for people who do not tend to fall asleep easily, while standing is usually suitable for people who are naturally meditative, that is, they enter a meditative state very easily. It is also suitable for people who are very experienced in meditation.

In any case, sitting is definitely the recommended position at the beginning – but sitting, reclining or standing must be comfortable. If you want to meditate in the "lotus position" – sitting with your legs crossed, your feet resting on your thighs – but it is uncomfortable, you should put this position off until you are sufficiently flexible. Rather make do with sitting in a comfortable cross-legged position or sitting on a comfortable chair, because otherwise all you will be able to think about during the meditation will be your aching legs. The same goes for people who suffer from back pains. First and foremost, see that you are comfortable.

Heightening Sexual Pleasure

During the first sessions of meditation practice, factors such as pain, tension, heat or cold (as a result of an unsuitable temperature) may hinder your entry into a meditative state.

In any case, you must perform the meditation in a quiet room. Sometimes, even in very quiet rooms, various sounds come in from the street or from the other rooms in the house. If you do not have the possibility of sitting in a completely quiet place, you must become accustomed to letting these noises simply flow past your ears. Don't try to ignore them – since the fact of ignoring them makes you concentrate on the sounds themselves – but rather know that they exist without concerning yourself with them at this moment. You can certainly be aware of them, but simply do not relate to them or pay attention to them.

The classic Oriental position for meditation is the yogi lotus, half lotus or sitting cross-legged. But again, these positions are not so essential to meditation and should only be used if they are really comfortable for you.

An equally acceptable method is sitting on a comfortably and upright chair with a good backrest, your back straight but not rigid, and your feet on the ground. The tip of your nose should be in a straight line with your navel, and your eyes should be gently closed.

The idea of transcendental meditation is to concentrate on one thing only. This can be a word or a combination of words that are called a "mantra," or an object such as a flower or a fruit.

This kind of meditation is known as transcendental meditation and is based, in part, on Indian practice. It was introduced to the West by Mahadishi Mahash Yogi, and gained a great deal of publicity in the 1970s because of the Beatles' interest in it.

Tantric Sex

In transcendental meditation, you repeat your mantra quietly to yourself over and over again. The mantra can be a totally meaningless word that is not meant to distract you from the meditation, and this is because the goal of the meditation is to empty your mind of thought completely.

A state of total non-thought can be a giant step forward for the Western person who hears and processes an enormous quantity of sounds and sights in one moment. (For instance, at this moment I am looking at a computer monitor; I am also aware of the white cup next to it, of the transparent yellow glass next to the cup, of the decorative blue tin box that contains pencils, and a number of other small objects in my range of vision. I hear two kinds of wind chimes outside my window, an airplane flying over, a neighbor speaking, a radio from another apartment, the hum of a ceiling fan, and the rustle of a sheet of plastic in the yard, moving in the wind. If I concentrate more, I can hear the hum of the refrigerator in the next room and a broader collection of sounds from the road. All these things – as well as odors and touch sensations – demand the attention of our nervous system all the time!

The fact that my attention was diverted from the focused task of writing by the noises, even for a few seconds, took its toll, and instinctively I went out into the yard to see what the strange sounds were – such as the knocking on the trashcan next to the gate of the house. Since detaching oneself totally from all thoughts is not that easy, the mantra focuses all the attention on itself. The fact that it is meaningless in that it does not evoke extensive associations causes it to become ordinary to the point of being a kind of "background hum" to the main issue: non-thought.

Some people use their own names, the name of someone

they know, a random name, or the name of some object that has no meaning for them. No, it is really not a good idea to use the name of your present or past girl/boyfriend, since this certainly does evoke associations. Since the name of a TV announcer is neutral (you don't feel anything personal toward him/her), it is much more suitable.

Of course, you can certainly invent words that are completely meaningless and do not have any deep feeling or emotion attached to them. The idea is that while you are repeating the word to yourself, your mind is emptying itself of thoughts, and in the end it will be impossible to think of anything else.

You may find that your mind loses its concentration and begins to think about something else, such as what they are cooking over there, what I will wear to the party tonight, I forgot to pick up the mail, I should do laundry now while the sun's shining – or whatever. If this happens (and it is far from rare), don't worry. Start to repeat the mantra to yourself again and enter the meditative state once more. Remain passive and maintain a relaxed approach toward any disturbance or distraction. If various thoughts come up in your mind, simply let them come and go, like those banners that are attached to planes that fly over the shore, or like an electronic message that comes and goes. It's there, you know, but there is no need whatsoever to devote any attention to it. Simply let it pass.

Another method is to concentrate on an idea, such as a mental picture, in the same manner. You can also retreat inward into your thoughts, and passively observe the passing thoughts without any criticism, comment or interference. The thoughts simply drift away, and you observe them and let them go on their way without criticizing them or relating to them. Another way is to close your eyes and simply hear the noise of external sounds without relating to them – but hearing them. They include all kinds of random noises such as cars, a kid yelling something, a radio, a neighbor or footsteps. Don't attribute any importance to these noises; don't define them or wonder what they are. It should be completely passive hearing, and you should not relate to it in any way. In fact, by directing the attention from the inside outward, a situation of non-thought or non-relating to oneself is created in a positive way. This is where the flow of relating to oneself stops (I want to eat. What's on TV? What she said isn't right. Grandma isn't feeling well. The neighbor is lovely, she brought food for the dog. What should I wear tonight? There's nothing in the closet. The temperature of the earth will rise by six degrees by the end of the century. The neighbors are doing home improvements again… and so on).

It does not really matter which method you choose to use. It's your decision, which suits and is based on your personality and feeling. However you do it, it is an intimate and important experience.

5
Breathing meditation

Another approach to entering a state of meditation is by means of creating a physical rhythm, such as by breathing. This seems to be the simplest of all the methods. In order to do so, breathe normally through your nose while focusing your mind on the sound and feeling of your breathing and on your rising and falling abdomen. Follow the rhythm of your breathing in your thoughts. If you are distracted by other ideas while doing so, don't worry – simply let them be drawn in and out of your head and try to restore your focus to the breathing. Don't force or compel yourself to concentrate – simply let it happen.

Ultimately, the meditation will become easy and automatic for you (like falling asleep). When the meditation time is up, take a deep breath, open your eyes, stretch, and slowly and gently return to your normal state. The ultimate goal is to discipline your mind so that it can concentrate on a single thing (or be in a state of non-thought). The deeper the concentration becomes, the more intense meditation process becomes.

6
Gazing at the sky

This is another meditation technique, and it is exactly like its name – gazing at the sky. Period.

Don't think about it, don't think about how it is, just do it. It makes no difference if the sky is blue, gray or bright and full of sunshine. That is unimportant. When you gaze at it, the idea is to leave everything else in your life behind until you feel that you are a part of the sky. When it happens, close your eyes, and you will almost certainly be able to see the picture of the sky you have just been gazing at in your mind's eye.

Another way to do this is by gazing at a candle. Light a candle and place it in front of you. Gaze at the flame and then close your eyes, and you will still be able to see the flame in your mind's eye.

Chapter 6

Starting alone, starting together

Know your body better
or
The beginning of intimacy

After you have made all the main preparations for making love, nothing can keep you from sexual enjoyment – after all, that is what you have been preparing yourselves for.

However, there is one more important element that can enhance your sexual pleasure.

Heightening Sexual Pleasure

1

Getting in touch with your personal enjoyment

Sexual enjoyment is an extraordinary thing. Nothing stresses this more powerfully than those moments in which you are learning to know your body intimately.

Focusing mainly on your sexual organs in front of the mirror, masturbate and try to understand what causes you the greatest pleasure during sexual arousal and orgasm.

Masturbation is not always considered to be desirable in the West, but according to tantric teachings, there is no better way of becoming familiar with your body than by masturbating. This is an extremely important point.

In other words, it is not possible to become an expert in the art of tantric happiness if you do not really know your body.

2

The tantrists believe that masturbation constitutes another aspect of the person's sexuality, and like any pleasurable experience of human sexuality, this too is a positive experience, and so it should be related to positively and openly.

Anything that is pleasurable is permitted, so there are many Eastern pictures of people pleasuring themselves, especially women.

Nothing enables you to know your body better than masturbation. Understanding the thing that gives you the greatest pleasure enables you to improve the quality of your orgasm, and also enables you to transmit it to your partner, so that he can also do it.

Another advantage of masturbation is that it usually improves the relations between the members of the couple. Through masturbation, the female partner can understand that she does not have to depend on her partner for her satisfaction and pleasure, and he, in turn, does not have to feel responsible for her pleasure. This will dispel a lot of tension he may feel and will place both partners on the same plane of pleasuring and feeling pleasure.

There are a lot of people who feel guilty about masturbating. According to the tantrists, these guilt feelings are completely unnecessary. There is nothing, absolutely nothing, wrong or bad about pleasuring yourself, and in any case, most people admit that they actually enjoy masturbating.

3
Female masturbation

The tantric masters suggest that the woman spread her legs in front of the mirror and look at herself. She should cover her body with massage oil and massage her body, passing her hands sensuously over every part of it, seeking areas that give her tremendous pleasure. These areas can be the sexual organs, of course, but some of them could also be other places such as the inner thighs and the inner arms. The tantrists believe that the entire body is an erogenous zone and that the arousal of any part of it can lead to sexual arousal.

Most of the attention should be focused on the genital region, which the woman should stimulate slowly, touching herself gently over the entire region, including the perineum (the area between the anus and the vagina) and the anus. She must experiment with various levels of pressure, light and strong, side to side and in circles.

When she brings herself to orgasm, she should hold her tongue against her hard palate. This is very important to the tantrists, because it completes the circle of sexual energy.

When the woman reaches a climax, she should also concentrate on her third eye chakra, which pulls the energy upward along the spine and through all the chakras into the top of her head.

This is an ancient tantric belief that is considered to be a tremendous act of spirituality. It is said that it raises the awareness to a great extent and also leads to a broader awareness.

4
Male masturbation

In the identical way, the tantric masters suggest that the man spread his legs in front of the mirror and look at himself. He should cover his body with massage oil and massage his entire body, using sensuous movements and searching for areas that give him tremendous pleasure.

Some of these areas may be self-evident, but others, such as the nipples, the inner thighs and the inner arms, may surprise him by the level of pleasure they provide.

The tantric masters believe that the entire body is an erogenous zone and that the arousal of any part of it can lead to sexual arousal. Now the man should focus on his genitals, including the scrotum, perineum and anus. He should experiment with various types of touch and various levels of pressure.

When the man reaches orgasm, he should hold his tongue

against his hard palate, as in female masturbation. This is very important to the tantrists, because it completes the circle of sexual energy. When he reaches a climax, he should, like the woman, concentrate on his third eye chakra, which pulls the energy upward along the spine and through all the chakras into the top of his head. As mentioned above, this is an ancient tantric practice that is considered to be an extremely spiritual act that also expands the awareness.

5
Masturbating in front of your partner

Masturbating in front of your partner is an especially loving thing to do. It is a way of sharing your most private and intimate sexual behavior, and it consolidates the channel of communication. It is also a way of showing your partner what pleasures you the most.

Prepare the setting beforehand, exactly as you would prepare it for making love, and sit opposite each other. Then begin to show each other (in turn) your genital region and how you like most to be touched.

You may prefer to do this together rather than in turn, so that neither one of you is "on display" and the experience will be a single and mutual one. In most cases, it is the first method that is likely to require deeper acquaintance and trust because of the innate fear that many people have of exposure and of total revelation.

6

Mutual masturbation

This is the last stage of sexual discovery, in which each partner in turn takes it upon himself to pleasure the other partner.

This stage may be the most difficult for many couples, since it involves a certain relinquishing of self-control. It is without a doubt worth doing, since it gives each partner a better understanding of what causes the other partner pleasure, and promotes confidence, trust, the bond and the openness between them. In certain relationships, this may serve as a quantum leap in their relationship in general. An experience like this creates a very tight bond of intimacy. But again, the experience must be reciprocal.

It would be a good idea to apply the same movements that your partner used on himself in order to satisfy and pleasure himself. It may not go completely smoothly the first time – few people manage it – but a certain level of practice is completely acceptable. You must both be prepared to help each other do things in the way you like. The simplest method is to tell your partner what you like, or make sounds of agreement and appreciation when you are touched in a pleasurable place, or adjust your position to something more pleasurable. In your turn, you must always pay attention to what your partner likes most.

Remember that this is a process of communication, so you must be prepared to listen to your partner carefully as well as to show him/her what is pleasant for you.

7
Massage

Touching is an extremely important sense, and without a doubt the star of the sexual context. It is something we learn from infancy, and it adds enormously to our ability to communicate as well as to our feeling of confidence as we grow up. When we reach adolescence, we tend to lose the use of touch somewhat, and this is a result of less sexual contact with one another.

Touch hints at a certain intimacy, and this is actually the reason that people sometimes find it difficult to touch people with whom they do not have intimate relations. It is worth emphasizing that touch is very important – not only in the sexual context, but also in the broader sense, since it is the most significant way of communicating with people. In other words, touch is always important, and it becomes more powerful when it exists within a sexual relationship in which it is considered to be the height of intimacy.

For this reason, because of awareness of the great importance of touch, massage is a very powerful and meaningful ritual for people who share it with each other. Massage is not only an excellent way of communicating with your feelings and transmitting them to your partner, but it is also a wonderful prelude to lovemaking. Massage soothes both body and mind, thereby encouraging the release of energy. As a result, the person is likely to feel aroused and relaxed at the same time, and also full of new energies.

When massage serves as a prelude to sex, you must use sensuous massage oil that enables your hands to slide easily over your partner's body.

Heightening Sexual Pleasure

There is a wide range of prepared massage oils on sale at cosmetic and aromatherapy stores, but you can also prepare massage oil yourself by adding your favorite essential oil to a vegetable carrier oil such as almond oil, grape seed oil or sesame oil. In principle, it is advisable to add one drop of essential oil to 2 cc of carrier oil (one drop to a teaspoon of oil).

Every essential oil has several properties that are unique to it. It is therefore a good idea to check that the oils are suitable for lovemaking, since they are absorbed by smelling as well as by penetrating the skin and then entering the bloodstream and the nervous system, where they may have a stimulating, invigorating, soothing or aphrodisiac effect.

The idea is that each of you performs the massage on the other one in turn. By means of the sensuous touch of your hands, you will cause your partner's body to relax, along with the possibility of the sexual arousal of both of you.

If the art of massage is new to you, pamper yourselves and go to a professional masseur who will demonstrate on your bodies how to give a pleasurable massage.

Pay attention to the feelings that are aroused in you, and then try to create the same feelings in your partner by performing those actions on his/her body. Ask your partner to speak to you during the massage and tell you what he is feeling. A massage is a pleasurable and enjoyable experience that is also supposed to stimulate passion. For this reason, you don't have to take the subject terribly seriously and learn all the rules of massage or begin to concentrate all your energy on releasing a stiff back by exerting massive pressure on certain points such as in deep muscle massage. Similarly, you don't have to "take your partner's body apart" by using the kind of massage that is applied to athletes. If you feel a tense point, simply continue massaging it gently, without using a great deal of strength, unless your partner asks you to do so. You must make sure not to press on the spine itself and not to use too much strength. Above all, the massage must be enjoyable, and it may be no less arousing for you if you let your fingertips feel your partner's pleasant skin and are mindful of his pleasure, since pleasure is certainly contagious.

Before beginning the massage, warm the oil up a little. Do this by standing the bottle (or the saucer of oil) in a bowl of warm water (without letting water get into the saucer!). It is important for your hands to be warm, too, since there is nothing relaxing about a pair of ice-cold hands on the body! Pour a little of the massage oil into one of your hands and rub your hands together.

Begin the massage with your partner lying face down on the bed. Rub the oil gently over your partner's back. Massage his upper back, neck, shoulders, lower back and buttocks, and then each leg and foot in turn. You must always work from the perimeters in the direction of the heart because this helps the blood enter the heart, thereby improving your partner's cardiovascular health. It also promotes a general good feeling.

After you have massaged the posterior side of your partner, he must turn over (ask him to do this in a gentle, calm voice), and now you can concentrate on the front part of his body: arms, hands, legs, face and scalp.

Chapter 7

Arousal

*Foreplay is an essential requirement for
lovemaking*

1
Foreplay

At this stage, you may already be prepared for
lovemaking. Foreplay is a stage that must not be skipped.
This is because good sex is not something rushed and hasty.
Moreover, only by means of sensitive and considerate
foreplay is it possible to be sure that both partners are
completely ready for intercourse, both physically and
psychologically.

In a clear and obvious way, the tantrists consider foreplay
to be an essential part of the ritual preparation for sex.
Foreplay has great significance in good sex, so it is
considered to be much more than merely sex. It could be
said that foreplay is an essential requirement for satisfying
lovemaking.

Sexual arousal is the first stage of lovemaking, and foreplay is the best, most certain and most enjoyable way of ensuring that arousal happens.

Foreplay is very important for the man because it enables him to get a strong erection that, of course, is essential before intercourse begins.

However, for the woman, foreplay is even more important, and that is because the woman takes much longer to become sexually aroused than the man. The woman must be sexually aroused so that her vaginal juices will flow properly during penetration.

The Eastern and Western approaches to foreplay are very different. In the West, foreplay is considered to be an addendum to intercourse, and it is often rushed through because not too much importance is ascribed to it. In the East, foreplay is considered to be an important and essential part of the entire sexual encounter. It gives both partners tremendous pleasure, especially the woman, even though it may not necessarily culminate in intercourse – this is especially true in the tantric belief.

2
The arousal of the woman

For a woman, foreplay is meant to be a long process that goes on for about 20 minutes and sometimes much longer. The best way of arousing a woman is by means of a long and concentrated series of movements.

It is best to begin by caressing her head and face, and then to move your hands slowly down her neck and shoulders until you reach her breasts. Any solid but gentle movement will work well, including caressing and massaging, as well as kissing and sucking the breasts and nipples. In a particularly orgasmic woman, this kind of foreplay can bring her to orgasm.

According to the Tantra doctrine, the entire body is an erogenous zone, not just the genitals. It is a good idea to remember this when you are devoting attention to as many other parts of the woman as possible. Add touch not just with your fingers, but also with other parts of your body, so that you create maximal contact with your partner. This should be extremely arousing, so it is worthwhile using your imagination and sensitivity in order to give the woman you love wonderful sensations.

Caress her belly, the inner parts of her arms and thighs, and gradually go over her entire body until you reach her genitals. Touch her vagina and her clitoris with your hands and your mouth and vary the type of pressures and movements.

Foreplay is not just a matter of arousal. It is also a wonderful method of communication between lovers who are mindful of each other's needs, so you should always try to respond to a touch that is nice for your partner and to her reactions, and do what she likes the best.

3
The kiss

Kissing is very important for the woman. Foreplay is not really perfect without a lot of deep and sensuous kisses. Many women in the West complain that the man does not invest enough time in kissing, and there is no doubt that the modern Western man can learn a great deal from the tantrists.

Tantric Sex

The tantric teachings recognize the importance of the kiss and even consider it to be an important part of lovemaking, almost like intercourse itself. Kissing is without a doubt a very intimate activity consisting of lips, saliva and tongues that create a deep, powerful and arousing bond between lovers.

The woman's upper lip is identified with her palate and clitoris, and for this reason, kissing or sucking it can have a very arousing effect for her. According to the tantric teachings, a relaxed mouth is much more sensitive than a nervous mouth, and they recommend open-mouthed kissing with eyes open. In this way, a meaningful exchange of visual contact can take place.

The tongue can both receive and give tremendous pleasure. It is wet and warm, strong and surprisingly flexible. Use it in any way you want, wherever the realms of desire and imagination take you, on your beloved's mouth, lips, tongue, tip of the nose or feet. As always, vary the rhythm, the speed and the pressure of the touch.

According to the tantric belief, the exchange of bodily fluids during lovemaking is very important, and the most important of all is the exchange of saliva. The tantrists believe that it is essential to show your partner love, trust and respect in order to taste their saliva, and when you try it, you will certainly want to do it again and again.

An aroused woman's saliva is known as "the jade fluid," and according to the tantrists, it is considered to be very beneficial for the man's strength and health. The tantrists claim that it is very important that when the woman reaches orgasm, she touches her palate with the tip of her tongue, since this completes the circle of sexual energy.

Accordingly, when the woman reaches her climax, she

must offer her tongue to her partner so that he can suck her saliva.

4
The man's arousal

It is much easier to arouse a man than it is to arouse a woman, but this does not mean that this should be done without sensitivity and imagination since – as many men will agree – there's foreplay that's OK, there's foreplay that's good, and there's foreplay that's outstanding, sensational. Your aim is always to give foreplay that's outstanding. Generally, the touch of the entire body arouses most men as well as the women who do it to them.

Touch many parts of your partner's body and let his reactions guide you, whether this is by him telling you or by his physical reactions. Vary the movements and the pressure of your touch.

Leave his penis until last, and wait until he is ready to be touched in that region. Don't worry, he'll let you know! Men generally like gentle arousal of the testicles and scrotum, and you can use your hands, your lips or your tongue for that.

5
Oral sex

One of the most powerful ways to arouse someone (of either sex) is by kissing, licking and sucking his/her genitals. This method is very intimate, and it provides extreme pleasure for both people, especially the passive partner. The tantrists rule that kissing, licking and sucking are highly effective in the process of sexual energy.

Fellatio, or oral sex with a man, can be done in a range of ways, according to the width of the open mouth and according to its wetness. Vary the oral movements, suck the penis along its length, and keep track of what is most pleasurable for your partner.

Cunnilingus, or oral sex with a woman, is sometimes the most effective way of arousing her. According to the tantrists, the vulva is the most sacred region of the woman's body and constitutes a symbol of life itself.

The man must kiss and lick her mound, run his tongue along it and between the external labia of the vagina. You can also put your tongue inside her vagina while making exploratory movements that can be deep or shallow, fast or slow, as you wish.

The clitoris is the woman's center of sexuality, and very often the woman enjoys it when the tongue goes over and around it. Sucking the head of the clitoris between your lips can have an almost magical effect, and often the result is orgasm, even in women who usually have a problem reaching a climax.

6
Mutual oral sex

The "upside-down" or "69" position is an effective way for both members of the couple to give and receive oral sex at the same time.

There are people who prefer to have oral sex in turns, and that is because it is not easy to muster the necessary level of concentration when they are both doing it at the same time. However, for others, the 69 position offers peaks of sexual pleasure.

Heightening Sexual Pleasure

According to the tantric writings, the perineum is the location of the root or base chakra, in which the dormant kundalini lies. A recommended tantric exercise is to place your tongue on your beloved's perineum, and then there is every chance that you will begin to feel tangibly the energy being aroused and uncurling up through the chakras. This can be done by both of you, to each other, when you are in the 69 position.

Chapter 8

Making love

Be mindful of pleasures…
There are always ways to do it better

1
Prolonging the ecstasy

However you do it, making love is one of the pleasures of life, and one of the most powerful experiences. It can never be bad, but there are always ways to do it better, and these require your attention.

However, don't let it stress you out. We are not talking about hard work, just about paying attention to the feelings of pleasure you experience. We are not referring to an experiment, that is, that you should try to pay attention to the feelings of pleasure you are having, since this effort is liable to jeopardize your enjoyment by interfering in the pleasure. It should happen naturally, especially if you feel comfortable and have an open attitude toward sex. Simply be mindful of the pleasures that are about to come – it won't just be fun, but it will also pay off.

2
Making love

Intercourse is the peak of sexual experiences. There are many wonderful ways of doing it, and people like different and varied positions.

Many people do not have one favorite position, but rather several different positions, according to their mood and the circumstances. The important thing is variety – a different position for every day of the week, perhaps – and keeping an open mind to a broad range of different and exciting positions. If you always made love in the same position, and closed your mind to trying out something new, sex would become boring and predictable.

3

The tantric approach to lovemaking is to encourage as much variety as possible, and to always be prepared to try something new as well as different approaches.

Experimentation and exploration in the sexual realm are always recommended, and if you are always willing to try out a range of pleasures and positions, you can keep your mind focused on the actual sex act itself.

According to the Kama Sutra – one of the most famous ancient tantric writings, the most refreshingly frank of all the erotic works ever written – there are actually very few basic sex positions. These are: the man on top, the woman on top, and the ones with rear entry. Everything else is actually a variation on one of the basic positions.

The Kama Sutra was collated into one work around about the fourth century AD, but it is surprising in its modern outlook, and we can all learn a great deal from it.

4
The man on top

The positions in which the man is on top of the woman are known by the name otana-bandha. These positions are actually preferred by many couples, and the reason for this could be that they permit full eye contact between the members of the couple, and this fulfills a powerful need for closeness and intimacy.

In tantric sex, maintaining eye contact is considered to be very important, because it consolidates and builds a very powerful communication between the couple, and also enables each of them to know what the other is thinking and feeling. Gazing gently and steadily into the other person's eyes works like a kind of sexual meditation that raises the sexual encounter to a higher plane. Moreover, the man-on-top positions permit an infinite range of kissing one's partner and of mouth kissing, which, according to the philosophy of tantric love, is well loved because of the intimacy and power inherent in it.

The man-on-top positions are especially well liked by men. This could be because they give the man full control of all the details of intercourse, such as depth of penetration and rhythm.

The most popular man-on-top position is the "missionary" position, in which the woman lies on her back with her legs apart. In the East, this position is called "the yawning position."

There are many possibilities for varying the missionary position, and these depend on what the woman chooses to do with her legs. This in fact is the main and important factor in changing the position.

For instance, the woman can pull her knees up toward her breasts and rest her feet on the man's chest. In this case, the position is called "the position of Indra's partner." Alternatively, she can wrap her legs around the man's back, and in this case the position is called "the position of the Lafita." Another possibility is for both partners to keep their legs straight, with one of them pressing his legs firmly along the outer part of the other's legs. This position is called "the pressing position." Another position entails the man lying in the other direction, his head facing the woman's legs, and in this case, the position is called "the position of the turn."

5
The woman on top

The positions in which the woman is on top of the man are known by the name poroshaita-bandha. These positions, like the man-on-top positions, permit full eye contact, which, as we mentioned above, increases intimacy. In tantric sex, eye contact is considered to be an especially important factor, because it creates a means for intimacy during sex itself. Here, too, the woman-on-top positions permit a broad range of kisses on the mouth, which are considered to be so important by the tantric sages.

When the couple have intercourse in this way, the woman has full control over the details of the act, such as the depth of the penetration and its rhythm.

The simplest and most widespread woman-on-top position features the woman sitting on top of her partner, facing him, her knees bent on either side of him. This position is known as "the position of the pair of tongs."

There are many ways of varying this position. The best known is when the woman sits in the opposite direction, that is, facing the man's feet. Another variation of the position is when the man sits cross-legged and the woman sits on him, her legs crossed behind his back. It is a good idea to stress that this position is considered to be particularly close and full of softness.

6
The "rear-entry" positions

When the woman assumes rear-entry positions, that is, when the man penetrates her when he is positioned behind her, it permits especially deep penetration, and this is a very good position especially if you are both in a very passionate mood. The couple can make love with rear-entry positions when they are lying down, standing, sitting or kneeling – since apparently this is the most passionate position of all. Lying next to each other in the "spoon position," with the man lying behind the woman, is a particularly serene and close position, in which both members of the couple enjoy a powerful feeling of union and intimacy.

7
Reaching orgasm

During sex, there are two particularly important things that make reaching orgasm easier for both parties. The first thing is breathing, and the second is pulling the pelvic floor muscles inward.

Breathing joins you to your sexual center, and so the more deeply you breathe, the closer you will be to your sexual energy.

Heightening Sexual Pleasure

Deep breathing intensifies your senses, thereby enabling you to feel your sexual responses more powerfully. It intensifies your pleasure and lets you understand your orgasmic potential.

Contracting the pelvic floor muscles (in a series of cyclical and rhythmic drawing-in movements) while making love helps increase the feeling of arousal. It helps the man delay ejaculation when he is close to orgasm – one of the fundamental principles of tantric sex. This action causes the woman's body to increase the blood flow to her genitals. In other words, it intensifies the sensitivity both in the vagina and in the clitoris.

Chapter 9

The orgasm

It is not the end but rather the beginning

1

According to the tantric writings, orgasm is not the end but rather the beginning, that is, it indicates a transition in focus from a physical experience to a profound spiritual experience. The orgasm builds a strong movement of sexual energy through the chakras – from the base chakra, which is located at the base of the spine, to the crown chakra, which is located at the top of the head – and in this way releases our spiritual focus.

This is the tantric view of orgasm, but even if you do not espouse the tantric philosophy, it is worthwhile checking out and studying anything that promises better orgasms, and many people – mainly women – report that the results are indeed worthwhile.

The tantrists consider the female orgasm and the male orgasm to be completely different.

They brought up the idea that the woman's orgasm is the more important one since it grants essential life forces, and for this reason, the woman's fulfillment is a very important goal to accomplish. The woman can reach orgasm over and over again, and even though she herself may have a kind of emission, it does not weaken her.

2

Many men will be surprised to hear that the male orgasm, according to the tantrists, is not a synonym for ejaculation, so in fact they can make love over and over (or for longer periods of time) and satisfy their female partner many times.

Men, as opposed to women, are weakened by ejaculation, so they have to try and avoid it unless they want to procreate (which is really the only reason for ejaculating).

3

The female orgasm

According to the tantric writings, the woman does not lose energy when she reaches orgasm – as opposed to the man. In fact, the situation is quite the opposite: women are thought to "gain" energy during sex because they absorb their partner's energy. In addition, repeated orgasms are thought to keep the woman fresh and young.

Perhaps that is the reason why masturbation was once thought to have an important advantage for women, and perhaps this fact explains why are so many ancient tantric pictures showing women pleasuring themselves. In almost total contrast to men, many women find it difficult to reach orgasm. This is therefore another reason why it is a good idea for women to masturbate in front of their partner, so that he can see exactly what he has to do in order to bring her to orgasm.

Women can experience different kinds of orgasms, such as the clitoral orgasm and the vaginal orgasm. Neither one is better than the other – they are simply different. Therefore, with the help of masturbation (either alone or in front of her partner), the woman can learn a great deal about how to reach orgasm. The tantrists called the clitoris various names such as "lotus bud" and "jade pearl." When the clitoris is stroked, flicked with a fingertip or pressed, it can bring the woman to orgasm.

On the other hand, the vaginal orgasm occurs as a result of internal stimulation, and it feels very different from the clitoral orgasm. Most women need a longer period of stimulation in order to reach a vaginal orgasm.

In addition to the clitoral and vaginal orgasms, there is the G-spot orgasm. Many people think that the G-spot is a new discovery, but in fact the tantrists were also aware of it, and they called it "the hidden jade moon" or "the heart of the lotus bud."

The G-spot is located at the entrance to the vagina, on its inner side. It is a small, slightly hard area as compared to the rest of the vagina. The man can stimulate the G-spot with his penis or fingers. It should be pointed out that a G-spot orgasm creates intense sensations of sublime pleasure.

4

The male orgasm

For the man, the orgasm constitutes the third stage in his sexual cycle. The three stages in the sexual cycle of the Western man are the arousal stage, when the man gets an erection; the plateau stage, when the man continues to be passionate, and the orgasm stage, usually when ejaculation occurs. After the last stage, the penis is flaccid and needs time to recover before it can "wake up" once more.

Things are different with the Eastern man. He does not relate to orgasm and ejaculation as synonymous, and he believes that orgasm should be something he can enjoy as many times as he wants, that is, without needing time to recover.

According to the tantric belief, semen contains vigorous life energy. For that reason, it must be conserved and not wasted, so the ability to reach orgasm without ejaculating is considered to be an essential sexual ability.

This may be surprising to the Western person, who generally believes that ejaculation is natural and healthy and constitutes solid proof of a man's masculinity and sexual prowess, so that nothing should be allowed to disrupt this process. However, in contrast to the prevailing opinion in the West, the ancient tantrists rule that orgasm without ejaculation, or "dry orgasm," enables the man to conserve his vitality.

They believe that controlling ejaculation will cause the man to be healthier and stronger, and as a result, to live longer. Similarly, controlling ejaculation, according to them, will cause the man's orgasms to be better, because they will become orgasms of his entire body, which are stronger and more pleasurable.

The idea is that the man will be able to experience multiple orgasms. As stated previously, the aim is not just better sex, but also a better and deeper relationship.

5
Controlling ejaculation

It sounds good; no more men who roll over after orgasm, depleted of energy, and fall asleep!

But how does he do it? The first step the man has to take in order to control his ejaculation is to be willing to discard all the notions he grew up with.

The man must forget all the nonsense about ejaculation being proof of his manhood and his sexual prowess. It isn't – it's simply an involuntary reflex. He must also be willing to jettison the idea that dominated the youth of many men – that ejaculation is a kind of sublime point, the peak of the sexual experience. In other words, the man must be willing to discard the entire notion of ejaculation, since it is certainly not the be-all and end-all of sexual pleasure! And it is in no way essential for sex.

Moreover, you (the man) will have to convince your partner about the wisdom of sex without ejaculation, since many women are just as guilty as men of turning ejaculation into a myth of the summit of the sexual experience. She must stop relating to ejaculation as a proof of the intensity of your feelings, or even of your love for her. Ejaculation is far from being a magical experience, and it is not ritual proof of what the man feels in his heart.

That's all a lot of mystical nonsense, and the woman must cooperate and understand this. She must understand and identify with you. After you have taken this step of self-understanding and of explaining to your partner, you have already gone halfway. Now you must redirect your sexual energies, concentrate on keeping them in your body, and from there transmit them to the woman you love.

It is not so complicated to refrain from ejaculating. It involves understanding how your body works – in other words, you must understand your sexual rhythms – what is the most powerful cause of ejaculation, which sexual positions are most conducive to ejaculation, and so on.

6
The male genitals

There are several things you can do in an attempt to control ejaculation. It is worth stressing that certain men may find one of the following methods satisfactory, while others should use a combination of the methods until they find the method that suits them. Don't expect to succeed first time round, and don't give up if you blow it every now and then. The process takes time, patience and practice, but if you believe in your ability to do it, you will almost certainly succeed.

Here, too, as with any other skill, the more you practice, the more you'll succeed. So don't be impatient – you'll get there in the end. Sex is a learning and teaching experience, and it is worthwhile learning the following ways and enjoying them.

Most Westerners tend to pamper themselves with sex only when in the grip of passion. However, the tantric teachings claim that it is preferable to set aside time and a place in which both members of the couple can practice what they have learned. By concentrating and practicing, the control of ejaculation will become easier to manage.

One of the things many men find helpful is to remain completely motionless. First concentrate, then relax every muscle in the genital area, including the anal muscles.

An important and helpful factor is pressing your tongue against your hard palate, about one centimeter behind your front teeth. You may find that this has a surprising and unusual effect that anchors you and helps you redirect your sexual energy downward, to the front of your body, to the base chakra (which is located at the base of your spine) where it comes from. The effect of this action will be to delay or stop ejaculation.

Take a series of deep and regular breaths. Their effect will be to slow down your heart rate, leading to a general slowing down of your body, and this will cause some kind of reduction in the urgent need to ejaculate.

Withdraw your penis slightly from your partner's vagina. This need not disturb or spoil intercourse because afterwards (when your need to ejaculate has decreased a bit) you can penetrate deeply again.

If the above methods are not good for you, it may be preferable for you to withdraw your penis from her vagina completely. Wait until you feel that you can resume without ejaculating.

Press your index finger and middle finger of one hand quite hard on your perineum, the area between the scrotum and the anus. This action will enable you to keep the semen in the prostate, where it will be reabsorbed into the bloodstream. When you're more experienced, you may even prefer your partner to do it. It will become a shared action for the two of you, and this is always good in sex.

Place your thumb on the inner part of your penis, with your index finger and middle finger on the upper side of the ridge of the glans, and press for about 10-15 seconds, until you lose the urge to ejaculate. You will almost certainly also lose your erection, but you will be surprised at how easy it is to get another one immediately. Your partner can use this pressing technique, if your prefer. Again, it is surprising how pleasant the joint attempt to control your ejaculation can be.

7
Orgasm of the entire body

After you have reached a state of controlling ejaculation skillfully, you must be able to use the combination of arousal, calming down and deep breathing that will enable you to achieve an orgasm of your entire body. This is definitely a climax that affects the entire body rather than just the penis area (that is, an orgasm that is felt only in the penis). This sensation is reported to be a more delicate feeling than a genital orgasm, and it is less intense and fast. In other words, it is not a momentary explosion of excitement, but rather a continuous and lengthy flow of pleasure.

8
Twilight time

After sex comes twilight time. This is the time for friendship, warmth and closeness. It is not the time to turn over and go to sleep. This is a special time, and it is important not to rush it. It is a time for lovers to enjoy each other while they are feeling completely relaxed and fulfilled both physically and emotionally.

Chapter 10

Tantric sex and Westerners

You want to improve your sex life

1

Tantric sex may not seem attractive to you at first sight. You may be skeptical. What chance is there that philosophical Tantra, ancient Eastern illumination, can help effect a change in the love life of sophisticated Western lovers? Is there any way of examining what the ancient tantrists – the supporters of the complicated tantric exercises surrounding the ancient Eastern art of lovemaking – had to say about the matter?

Yes, it may look like a spurious suggestion, but be patient. It is not easy to extract the true essence of sexual happiness from the words of the Tantra sages and make them accessible to modern lovers who are always on the lookout for things that produce good sex, better sex, and even better sex.

Surprisingly, this is not a load of nonsense. These are understandable and accessible teachings about sexuality, and it is astounding just how comprehensible, clear and logical they are to many people.

2

It is worthwhile stressing that no matter what your interest in Eastern philosophy and spirituality may be, there is every chance that you want to improve your sex life. Most people want to. Many of us go a long way in order to achieve this, and if making the acquaintance of the words of the sages from thousands of years ago offers you a path to sexual happiness, there is no real reason for you not to try it!

The essence of sex, according to the tantric philosophy, is the use of sexual intimacy as a tool for increasing, improving and discovering your spiritual pleasure. You and only you are responsible for your sexuality and your spirituality, and the two are intricately intertwined. In other words, you and only you can change things.

The tantrists consider sex to be a completely normal activity – which it is. Few people will dispute this. However, the tantrists took the subject one step further. They also believe that something that is natural cannot be bad. Nevertheless, it is doubtful that everyone would agree with this declaration.

The only kind of sex that was considered bad by the tantrists is unsatisfying sex, and there is no doubt that to view sexuality in this way is a very modern view. It is a view that does not seem strange or unusual to most people nowadays. It is worth stressing, claim the Tantra sages, that sex that is performed without the full and true consent of both parties, or as a result of some kind of manipulation and not out of emotional cleanliness, is not considered to be "sex" at all. It is so despicable, in their eyes, that it is not even worthy of being included in the definition of "sex", which, as we have said, the tantra sages held in such high regard.

3

According to the tantric philosophy, any kind of sexual experience is permissible. The only accusation (which is justified) that can be leveled at sex is when it is put at risk it by faking, or when the potential for sexual experience is wasted. Sex is considered to be an opportunity to learn, and the opportunity to increase your sexual experience is always good. If, in addition, sex also causes you pleasure, so much the better.

Anything that gives you pleasure is healthy and good for your physical and mental health. (Of course, everything must be in proportion; taking anything to extremes is not effective.) As such, sex is always supposed to be an exciting and uplifting experience.

4

In the tantric belief, there are no rules relating to the question of whether sex must only occur in the framework of marriege, or whether extramarital sex is wrong. However, while the question of marriage is not considered essential, the advantages of sex within a loving and stable relationship are considered to be manifold. All the tantric texts stress this clearly. Sex without a loving context is considered to be "second-rate" sex.

It would be a mistake to think that Tantra advocates engage in a great deal of sexual activity. This is wrong. In fact, the opposite is truer. Tantra's starting point has surprising moral depth. The tantrists would say that good sex requires time and practice – that is, practice with the same person. In order to be good lovers, something we all want, we have to recognize the needs of our lover and the things that are important to him/her. And this can't happen overnight, of course.

For this reason, this belief indicates that the tantrists would be shocked at the idea of a one-night stand. Sexuality is the distribution of sexual energy, and you cannot achieve this if you are only having sex for the sake of sexual release. "Selfish sex" is a contradiction in terms, and it is certainly not good sex. Love, according to most of the tantric texts, is one of the most powerful energies that the human being can experience. Love, like sex, is supposed to be channeled in order to further the person's spiritual experience.

5

Tantric sex, like many new ideas, can offer you a completely new way of thinking, and as such, the idea and the perception may not be easy for Westerners to understand, let alone assimilate into their lifestyles. Many people latch on to the idea almost instinctively, while other people find it a repugnant suggestion that requires a fundamental change in belief. This attests to the fact that the process may be much harder and much longer.

Even for those who link up to the idea quite easily, tantric sex is not devoid of difficulties, since it is an extremely complex topic. It means being prepared to challenge beliefs that you may have held for many years and to which you are very attached, sometimes without even thinking.

There are few people who do not have a problem with breaking old habits. There is no doubt that it is difficult to do so, so don't allow yourself to give up because of your doubts. Hesitation is human and shows that you don't rush into things without thinking about them, which can only be good. Thousands of people have succeeded in getting beyond this point and achieving tremendous things. For this reason, muster courage and trust yourself, since you too can do it.

6

The first and most essential thing that human beings are supposed to do when seeking sexual happiness is to take responsibility for their sexuality. They must accept the fact that they and only they are responsible for their own enjoyment from sex.

As we said above, this step is basic and essential, so you have to understand that only you can achieve it. You must believe in it, and you must believe in yourself. No one else is responsible for your sexual happiness – only you.

This may sound obvious, and you may even think that there is no point to this declaration, but it is worthwhile stressing that not everyone thinks or believes it. In fact, many people discover that it is surprisingly difficult for them to accept the fact that realizing their sexual potential is their responsibility. Similarly, many people have never even thought about it, and fewer have ever done anything significant in that respect.

Heightening Sexual Pleasure

Most people assume that their sexual happiness is their partner's responsibility. It should be mentioned that this assumption is made mainly by women. If a woman does not succeed in reaching orgasm during intercourse (or if it is difficult for her), she is liable to quickly jump to the conclusion that it is her partner's fault. However, this is not the case, and so it is important – very important – for the woman to understand that this matter depends on her alone.

This is not just essential, but also very exciting, because it means that the potential of each person to reach sexual orgasm depends only on him.

It is important and also very desirable to think positively, and it turns out that this is the most essential thing you can do for yourself. Never doubt your ability to achieve orgasm and consequently to achieve sexual happiness. This may sound too simplistic, but thinking positively about this topic as well as having faith in your ability to achieve orgasm is very important.

7

A lot of people, especially women, have had unpleasant or painful sexual experiences, and have discovered the world of sex from an atmosphere of oppression and prohibition. It is also possible that various other problems caused them to believe profoundly (sometimes unconsciously) that they would never achieve orgasm. This belief itself – especially when it is below the surface and the person is not aware of it – is liable to be destructive, and so it is necessary to work consciously at changing this negative pattern of belief and thinking.

8

Beyond this crucial and important belief, it is a really good idea to devote the necessary time and space to yourself in order to discover exactly what you have to do.

The most difficult part is taking the first and vital step of committing yourself to the steadfast (non-compromising) approach, which states that your sexual happiness depends on you alone. If you have succeeded in opening this gate and going through it, walking along the paths of Tantra will be easier.

As we said previously, in order to achieve the experience of tantric sex, you have to come with a positive approach as well as (and mainly) with a true desire to enjoy yourself.